Contact Lens Primer

Contact Lens Primer

Monica Chaudhry
BSc (Hons) Ophthalmic Techniques
Dr RP Centre for Ophthalmic Sciences
All India Institute of Medical Sciences
New Delhi

JAYPEE
JAYPEE BROTHERS MEDICAL PUBLISHERS
The Health Sciences Publisher
New Delhi | London

Jaypee Brothers Medical Publishers (P) Ltd

Headquarters
Jaypee Brothers Medical Publishers (P) Ltd
23/23-B, Ansari Road, Daryaganj
New Delhi 110 002, India
Phone: +91-11-23272143, +91-11-23272703
+91-11-23282021, +91-11-23245672
E-mail: jaypee@jaypeebrothers.com

Corporate Office
Jaypee Brothers Medical Publishers (P) Ltd.
4838/24, Ansari Road, Daryaganj
New Delhi 110 002, India
Phone: +91-11-43574357
Fax: +91-11-43574314
E-mail: jaypee@jaypeebrothers.com

Overseas Office
JP Medical Ltd
83 Victoria Street, London
SW1H 0HW (UK)
Phone: +44 20 3170 8910
E-mail: info@jpmedpub.com

EU GPSR Authorised Representative
Logos Europe, 9 rue Nicolas Poussin
17000, La Rochelle, France
Phone: +33 (0) 6 67 93 73 78
E-mail: Contact@logoseurope.eu

Website: www.jaypeebrothers.com
Website: www.jaypeedigital.com

Inquiries for bulk sales may be solicited at: jaypee@jaypeebrothers.com

Contact Lens Primer

First Edition: **2007**

Reprint: **2025, 2026**

ISBN 978-81-8061-932-8

Typeset at JPBMP typesetting unit

***Printed** at:* **Sterling Graphics Pvt. Ltd. India**

Om Sai Ram

To
my parents, my husband and my son
who
supported me for this academic exercise

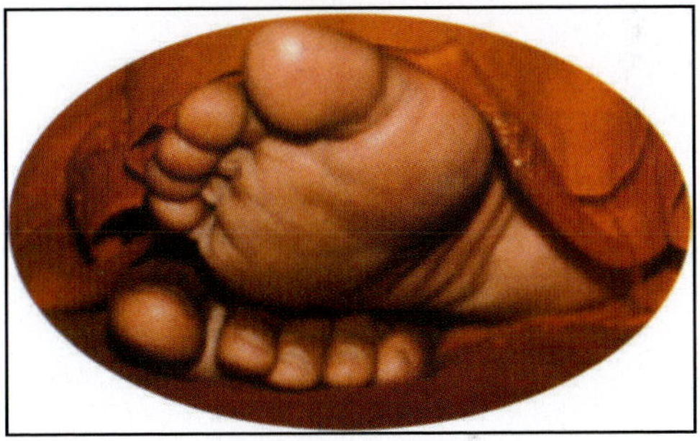

Preface

For several years I have been attempting to introduce students to comparatively easy technique of fitting contact lenses. During this period I have been unable to recommend a textbook that deals with the subject quickly and simply and yet is sufficiently comprehensive.

This book is an attempt to supply such a manual.

This little book not presume to tell the student all that he/she needs to know about contact lens, for which there are many larger books available. This book aims to decongest the contact lens curriculum for the students.

The intention of this book is also to guide contact lens practitioners who have not had any formal training in contact lens fitting. For them I have attempted to keep the language simple.

I am aware of many inadequacies and omissions and have avoided undue details and views. If the students find these notes more readable it will be justified.

It is hoped that it will enable the beginners to acquire a rapid but thorough grasp of a sophisticated yet simple discipline.

Monica Chaudhry

Acknowledgments

I wish to place on record the invisible hand of, IACLE—International Association of Contact Lens Educators, behind this project. They are doing services to all contact lens educators globally by improving their knowledge, providing resources, and upgraded the standards of contact lens fittings not only in my country but also all over the world. It is with their guidance and support that I am able to share my knowledge with my fellow practitioners across the country. IACLE resources have answered countless questions about topics where the knowledge surpassed mine. I am indebted to the IACLE organization, especially Prof Brien Holden and Debbie Sweeney and Lakshmi Shinde for their support and encouragement.

It is not possible to acknowledge everyone who helped me write this book but special mention is due to Prof VK Dada, my first teacher and guide; Prof JS Titiyal who is not only a good surgeon but also a great teacher as well; Prof S Ghosh who has always been encouraging and permitted me to write this book and Dr Namrata Sharma who was the first to convince me that I could accomplish the task.

It is also great pleasure to acknowledge my indebtedness to Mr Harminder Singh for the photographic work; to Ms Shivani Chawla for turning my amateur sketches into useful illustrations and for all the artwork; to Ms Sudha for assisting me in recording patients' slit-lamp photographs. Last but not the least I thank all my students and colleagues who have stimulated me with encouragement and criticism.

I am grateful to M/s Jaypee Brothers Medical Publishers (Pvt) Ltd., New Delhi whose gracious cooperation, jet propelled the text toward completion of production.

Above all, I am indebted to my family who did what families do best-care.

The International Association of Contact Lens Educators (IACLE), an organization sponsored by the international contact lens industry, developed some of the material included in this book. IACLE encourages the use of its material (resources) so that others may benefit from its endeavors.

The supply of this material and permission to use it is gratefully acknowledged.

Contents

1 Contact Lens Milestone

1508	Leonardo de Vinci described contact lens.
1845	John Herschel—theoretical application of CL.
1888	Adolph Fick—used glass shells on rabbit corneas. Trials using glass as lens material.
1934	PMMA material patented—John Crawford and Rowland hill. Development of PMMA material
1937	CAB lenses.
1948	Kevin Tuohy—12 mm corneal lenses.
1954	Experiments on HEMA lens material by Otto Witchterle and Drahoslav Lim.
1961	HEMA patented.
1970	Hydrogels era—rapid developments in designs.
1972	First RGP lens—silicon acrylates.
1981	First cosmetic extended wear (HEMA)
1984	Disposable lenses (Orlando Battista—gave the concept of 1st collagen lens).
1989	Hybrid—soft perm lenses.
1994	Daily disposable lens. Newer and newer designs of hydrogels—toric/bifocal/multifocals.

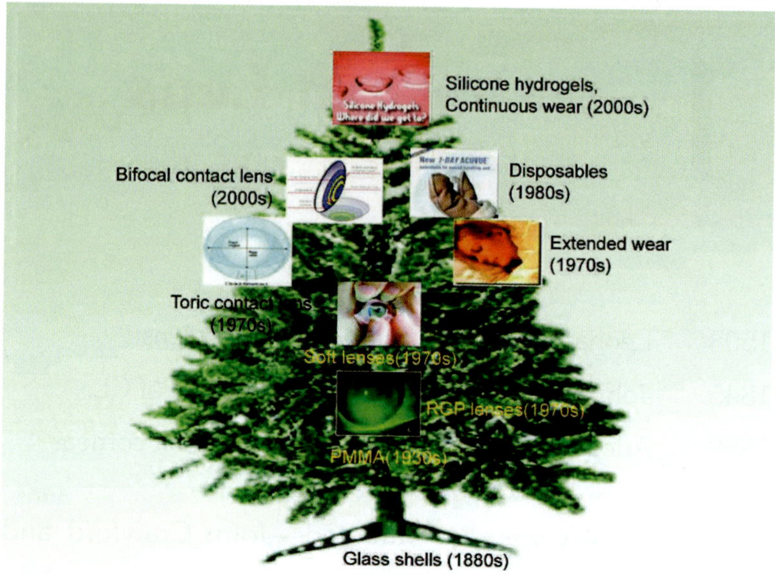
Silicone hydrogels,
Continuous wear (2000s)
Bifocal contact lens
(2000s)
Disposables
(1980s)
Extended wear
(1970s)
Toric contact lens
(1970s)
Soft lenses(1970s)
RGP lenses(1970s)
PMMA(1930s)
Glass shells (1880s)

Fig. 1.1: Tree of contact lens

2000 Continuous wear lens material—Siloxane containing hydrogels.

2 Contact Lens Terminology

Before proceeding further, it is necessary to define terms used to describe the form and dimensions of corneal contact lenses. These may vary in different countries.

Some Basic Definitions

1. **Blank** or the button from which the rigid or a soft lens is fabricated by lathe (Fig. 2.1).
2. **Semi finished blank**—A blank where base curve is pre-generated.

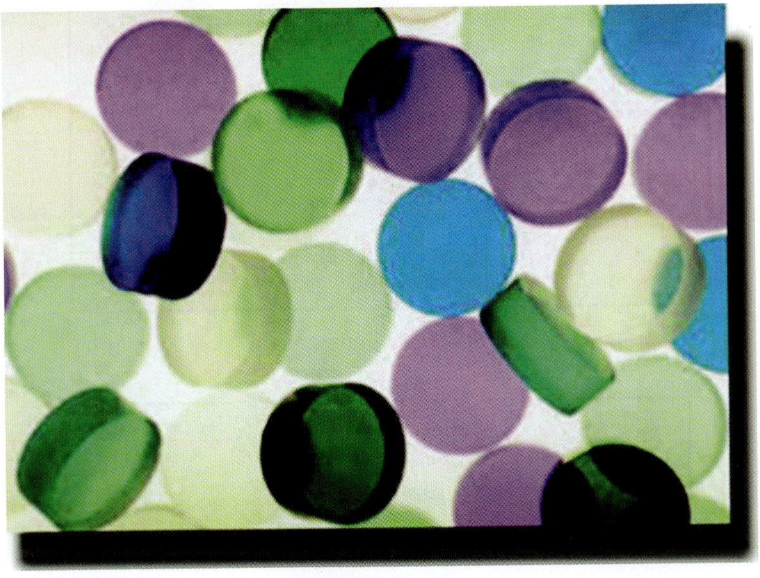

Fig. 2.1: Blank

3. **Semi finished lens**—A lens that has the back and the front curve cut. The peripheral curves and the edge is not yet fabricated.
4. **Finished lens**—A lens ready to be worn on the eye.

The Overall Contact Lens has Following Key Design Features (Figs 2.2A and B)

1. Base curve
2. Power
3. Lens diameter
4. Peripheral curves
5. Optic zone
6. Central thickness
7. Edge design.

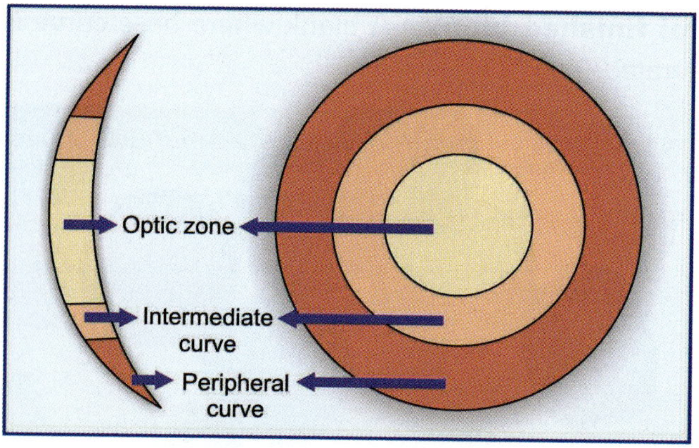

Fig. 2.2A: Lens zones

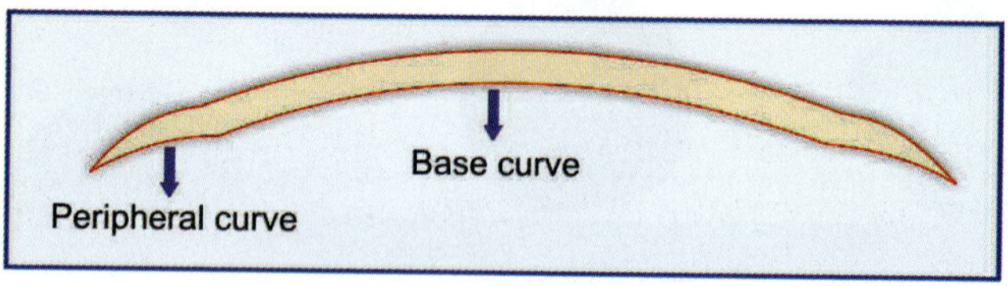

Fig. 2.2B: Overall lens design

Base Curve (BC)

Base curve or BC is also called as BOZR—Back optic zone radius, BCOR—Back central optic radius or CPC—Central posterior curve.

This is the back curve of the contact lens, which contours the front surface of the eye. To achieve a proper fit the base curve of the contact lens should be aligned with the curvature of the cornea.

Base curve is expressed in mm (millimeters) or diopters.

Example—8.1 mm, 8.3 mm. 8.6 mm, etc.

Also 8.1 mm is a steeper base curve than 8.3 mm, and 8.3 mm is steeper than 8.6 mm. So a longer base curve produces flatter base curves.

In diopters 44.0 D, is said to be steeper than 41.0 D radius of curvature.

Base curves can be **spherical or aspheric.** An aspheric base curve as the name suggests flattens from center to periphery and matches the corneal asphericity.

The apshericity is specified by e-value. Following are the e-values and their shape correlation:

e-value	*shape*
Zero	spherical
Between 0-1	elliptical
1.0	parabolic
> 1.0	hyperbolic

Most aspheric contact lenses have e-values from 0.3 to 1.1. Larger e-values are fitted in multifocal designs.

Since the base curve in case of aspheric lenses varies from center to periphery, the base curve of the aspheric lens is denoted as PAR-posterior apical radius which is a single point curve of the geometric center of the lens. This has little significance as value because the fitting will depend upon the ultimate design and shape of the back curve.

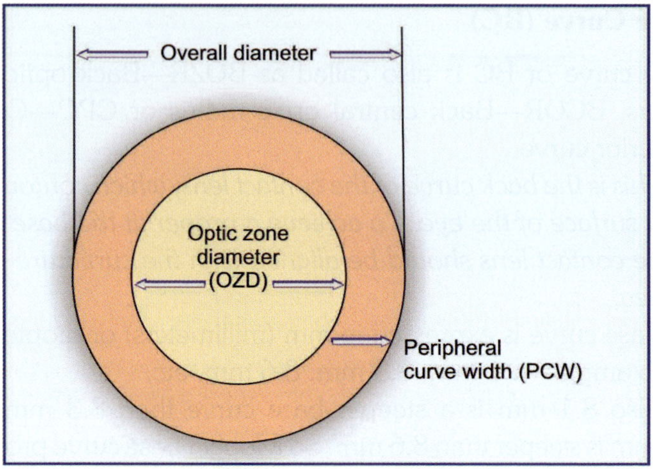

Fig. 2.3: Optic zone diameter/overall diameter

Overall Diameter (OD) (Fig. 2.3)

The length of the lens across its widest diameter is called the overall diameter or the lens diameter.

It is specified in millimeters. A soft lens is usually 12-15 mm and a rigid lens is of 8 to 10 mm diameter.

Diameter depends upon the corneal diameter and the palpebral aperture. Larger the corneal diameter greater is the overall diameter of the lens required.

Peripheral Curve/Curves (Fig. 2.4)

- A lens with a single base curve is called a Monocurve Lens.
- A lens with two curves at the back is called a Bicurve lens.
- A lens with three curves is called as a Tricurve lens.
- A lens with more than three curves is called a Multicurve lens.

So a Monocurve lens will have one base curve and no peripheral curve. A Bicurve lens will have 1 base curve and 1 peripheral curve. A tricurve lens will have 1 base curve and 2 peripheral curves and so on.

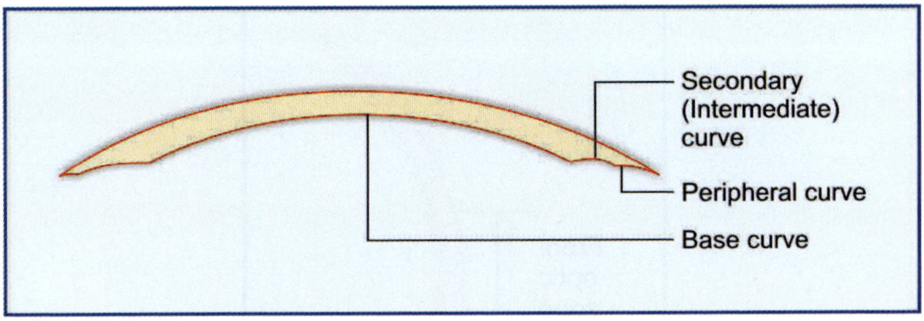

Fig. 2.4: Peripheral curves of a tricurve lens

The peripheral curve or PC is the curve surrounding the base curve on the posterior surface of the lens. If there is more than one peripheral curve then the inner curves are called **secondary or intermediate curves.**

PC is also alternatively called as PPCR – posterior peripheral curve radius.

The peripheral curves are flatter than the base curve, and the peripheral most curves will be the flattest one in a normal contact lens design, which is done to match the corneal shape.

Bevel /Blend

The junction between the base and the peripheral curves are blended properly to give a smooth transition and junction. Blending is the smoothening of the junction of the base curve and the peripheral curves. A well-blended junction is important for the comfort of the lens. Blending is soft, medium or heavy.

Peripheral Curve Width

The peripheral and the intermediate curve have a fixed width or size. It is usually 0.3 to 0.5 mm wide. It depends upon the optic zone diameter and the overall diameter.

Optic Zone (OZ) (Fig. 2.5)

The central optic portion, which carries the base curve of the lens, is called the optic zone. It is the central circular portion of

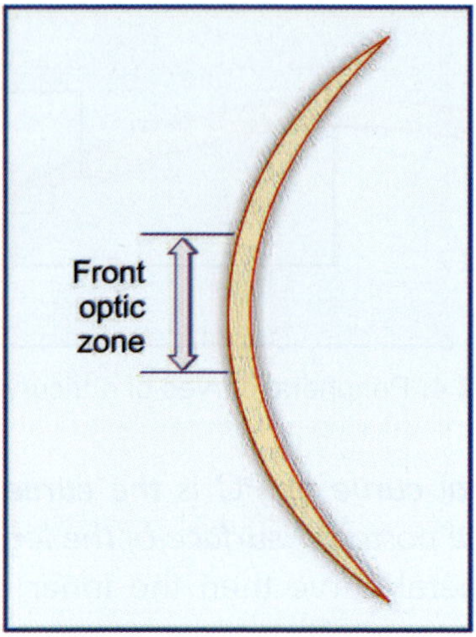

Fig. 2.5: Front optic zone

the lens where the power of the lens is located. The optic zone should cover the pupil properly both in scotopic and mezopic condition of light to avoid glare and flare problems.

The average size of the optic zone is 7 to 8.5 mm in case of rigid lenses and 7 to 12.0 mm in case of soft lenses.

Optic Zone Diameter (Fig. 2.3)

It is the diameter of the optic zone specified in millimeters. It is also the overall diameter minus the peripheral curve width.

Power

The power of the lens is ground on the front surface of the lens. A plus lens will be thicker in the center and the minus lens will be thicker in the periphery.

Central Thickness

It is the center thickness of the contact lens or the distance between the anterior and the posterior surface of the geometric center of the lens usually specified in millimeters.

Center thickness has its impact on fitting. The thickness of the lens also affects the oxygen transmissibility. Each lens material has its critical thickness, reducing beyond that leads to flexure problems.

Single Cut vs Lenticular Lens Design

Single cut design is the lens design, which has a single continuous curve in the front. The back surface is either monocurve (with single curve), bicurve (with two curves—base curve and peripheral curve), tricurve (with three curves—base curve, intermediate curve and peripheral curve) or multicurve (base curve and more than 2 peripheral curves).

A lenticular design is a lens designed with the optically powered portion of the front surface confined to the middle of the lens surrounded by the peripheral portion. In this case the front optic zone diameter is reduced and a front peripheral curve or curves are added. The portion of the lens- which does not carry the optic zone, is called the carrier. It is just like a spectacle lenticular designed lens.

Lenticular lens reduces the thickness of the lens and thus provides greater comfort and improves the transmissibility.

Lenticular design is commonly made in high-powered lenses.

Sagittal Depth: Sag (Fig. 2.6)

Sagittal depth or Sag is the perpendicular distance between the geometric center of the back of the lens surface and the diameter of the lens.

Sag values have their importance in fitting soft contact lenses. *The lens with a greater sag value will behave steeper than the lens with the lesser Sag.*

Sag values are dependent on the diameter and the curvature.

If the diameter of the lens is kept constant increasing the base curve radius decreases the sag or flattens the lens. Let us suppose there are 2 lenses of same 14 mm diameter, and if the

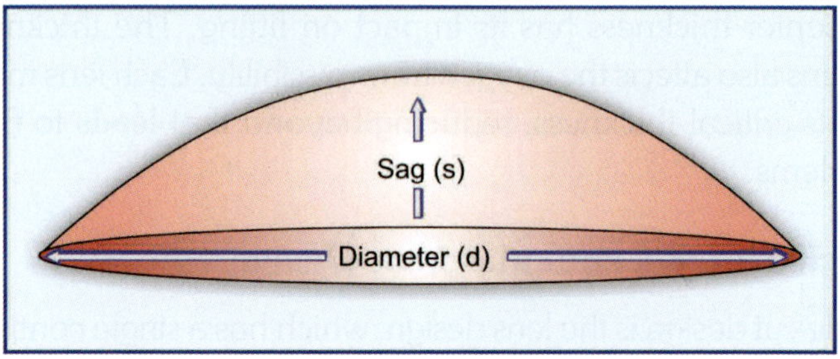

Fig. 2.6: Sagittal depth

radius of curvature is increased from 8.3 to 8.6 the lens with 8.6 mm radius will have lesser Sag or will behave flatter. Similarly if the base curve is kept constant and the diameters are changed, the lens with smaller diameter will have lesser Sag or will behave flatter (Fig. 2.7). Suppose there are 2 lenses with 8.6 BC but one lens has a diameter of 13.0 mm and the second lens has a diameter of 14 mm. The 13 mm lens will have lesser Sag.

Increasing the sagittal height tightens the lens, which can be done by either decreasing the base curve or by increasing the diameter.

Edge Lift (Fig. 2.8)

The terms axial edge lift (AEL) and the radial edge lift are used to describe the distance between the lens and the cornea for each of the lens zones (Fig. 2.9).

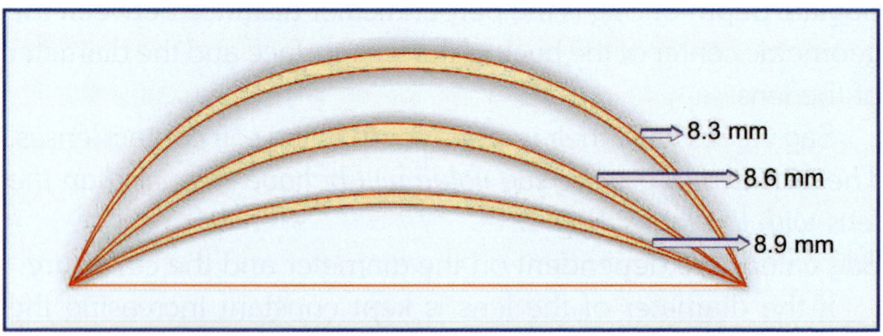

Fig. 2.7: Different base curves give different Sag provided diameter is same

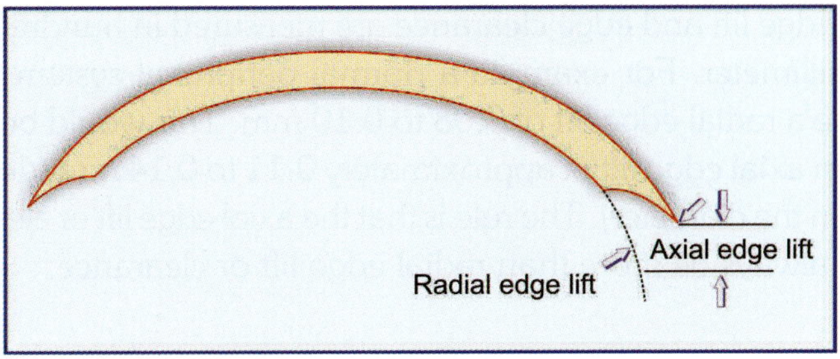

Fig. 2.8: Axial edge lift and radial edge lift

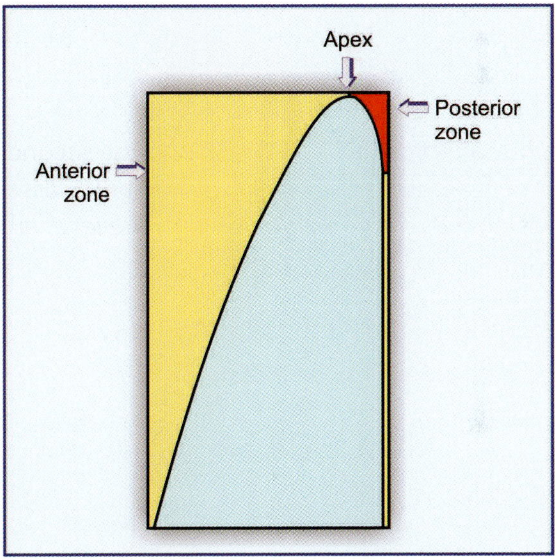

Fig. 2.9: Lens edge zone

AEL is the distance between the apex of the lens edge and the continuation of the base curve, measured parallel to the lens axis. REL is the distance between the apex of the lens edge and the continuation of the base curve.

Edge clearance, is the distance between the peripheral curves highest point (the lens apex edge) and the peripheral cornea.

Edge lift and edge clearance are measured in hundredths of a millimeter. For example a normal peripheral system would have a radial edge lift of 0.08 to 0.10 mm. This would be equal to an axial edge lift of approximately 0.11 to 0.14 mm (depends upon the diameter). The rule is that the axial edge lift or clearance will always be more than radial edge lift or clearance.

3 Contact Lens Design

Design of the contact lens is an important issue because it optimizes the ocular response for the individual and the population at large. The purpose is to achieve comfort, safety and vision. The design of the RGP lens can be more complex than the soft lens.

Soft Contact Lens Design

The design of the soft contact lens depends upon the following parameters of a soft lens:

1. Diameter
2. Thickness
3. Curvature—front and back

   With thin flexible lenses design is almost irrelevant.

Back Surface Design

1. Monocurve—Usually are not made in monocurve designs (Fig. 3.1).
2. Bicurve—Common, an central optic zone design and one peripheral curve.
   - PC—0.8 to 1 mm flatter
   - Width—0.5 to 0.8 mm.
3. Multicurve—Lenses, which have many curves, flexible lenses don't need a multicurve design.
4. Aspheric—Shapes cornea better, fewer base curves need to be made with aspheric back curve design, it is difficult to manufacture (Fig. 3.2).

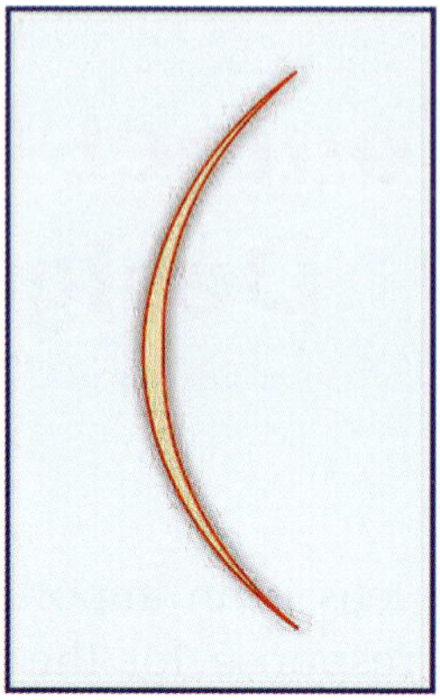

Fig. 3.1: Monocurve design

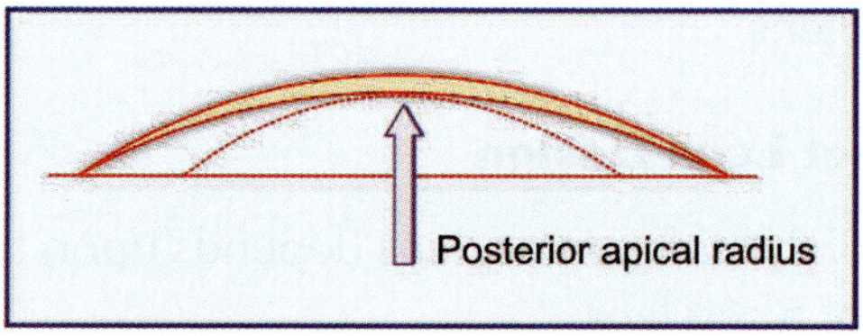

Fig. 3.2: Aspheric lens back curve

Front Surface Design of Soft Contact Lens

It is the front surface design that contains the front optic zone depends upon the power. The front design varies in bifocals/ multifocals.

Edge of Soft Contact Lens

The edge has a little effect than rigid lenses as it is mostly under the lid. Yet, thick is less comfortable and a very thin lens edge can cause mechanical cutting.

Manufacturing Technique and Design

There are three main techniques of soft contact lens manufacturing, different techniques create different designs like:

- A soft contact lens made with lathe is used to create simple designs.
- The spin technique creates simple back surface designs.
- The mould (– wet –) has very little limitation in making variation in designs.
- The spin + lathe or mould + lathe have same limitations as lathe.

Rigid Gas Permeable Lens—Design

The ultimate goal of the rigid lens design is to achieve ideal fit, which can be discussed in later chapter.

- Center—alignment.
- Mid peripheral—align with minimum clearance.
- Peripheral curves—0.3 to 0.5 mm wide.
- AEL (axial edge lift)—75 to 100 μ clearance.

The design of rigid lenses is very essential for fitting. They can be bicurve, tricurve or multicurve.

The **back surface design** of the rigid lens can be:

1. Spherical—gives better vision and centration.
2. Aspheric—Better alignment but more difficult to manufacture, is also difficult to verify, and leads to greater decentration.

Optic Zone and the Diameter

The size of the optic zone should be larger than the pupil size and it should cover it during the movement. The optic zone is also dependent upon the overall diameter and the peripheral curves.

The optic zone and the diameter have a direct correlation in RGP lenses.

The average size of the lens diameter is 9.2 to 9.4 mm.

One must select a small diameter lens (8.8 to 9.0 mm) – if the pupil size is small, or the corneal curvature is steep(> 45.0 D) or if the palpebral aperture is small.

The large diameter lens (9.6 to 9.8 mm) is selected in large pupils (> 8 mm) or flat corneas (< 42.0 D) or large palpebral apertures.

The optic zone size is also dependent on power. Higher the power smaller is the optic zone.

Edge and Edge Design Position (Fig. 3.3)

Edge is very important factor in giving comfort in RGP lenses. Lenses with rounded edges are most comfortable. This is because the anterior surface of the edge interacts with the lid, which is the main cause of sensation to the wearer. If the edge profile is rough or square at the anterior side the lens will be least comfortable, whereas the posterior design even if is square, the lens will be comfortable.

Center Thickness (CT) (Fig. 3.4)

The new generation rigid lens materials are softer and have some flexure more so on astigmatic corneas. This flexure is because of the pressure of the upper lid on the lens. Each lens material has a *Critical thickness*. This critical thickness is the minimum central thickness which can be made of a particular lens material so that the lens does not flex on the eye. If the astigmatism is more than 1.50 diopters increase the center thickness to avoid flexure. Central thickness is also more in higher Dk lenses.

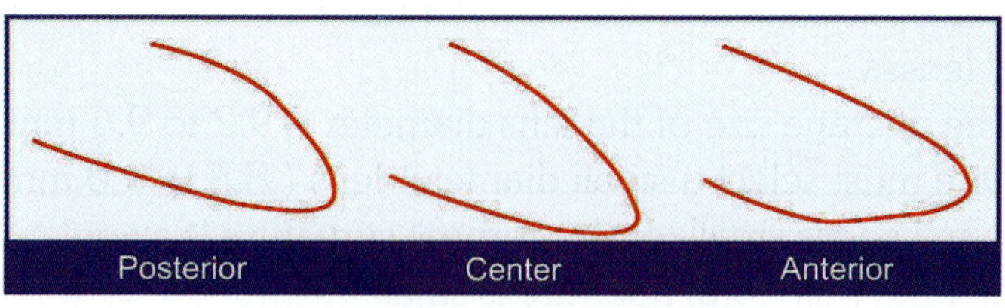

Fig. 3.3: Edge design/profile

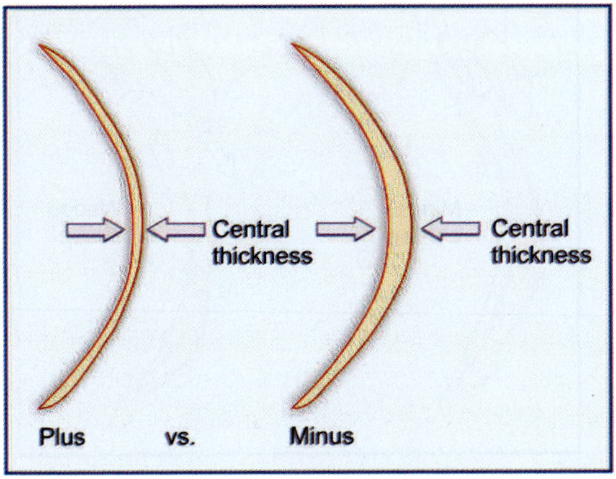

Fig. 3.4: Central thickness of plus vs minus lens

Front Surface Design

The front surface design of the rigid lens is dependent upon the power or the BVP (back vertex power) of the lens.

Sometimes, especially in higher powers, to achieve a proper centration the lens front surface design is made in lenticular form. The lenticulation reduces the centre thickness and mass in high plus powers, and also improves the oxygen transmissibility.

In combination with lenticulation the lens edge can be made to have a **minus carrier** to improve the interaction with the lid. By adding a minus carrier the lens is lifted up by the lids and reduces the lid interacting specially in high powers. Plus lenticulation is used in high minus lenses and minus lenticulation is used for all plus lenses (Fig. 3.5).

The Center of Gravity and the Design

The contact lens will be more stable and comfortable if the center of gravity is posteriorly located. The anterior location of center of gravity leads to a dislocated or low riding lens. The design of

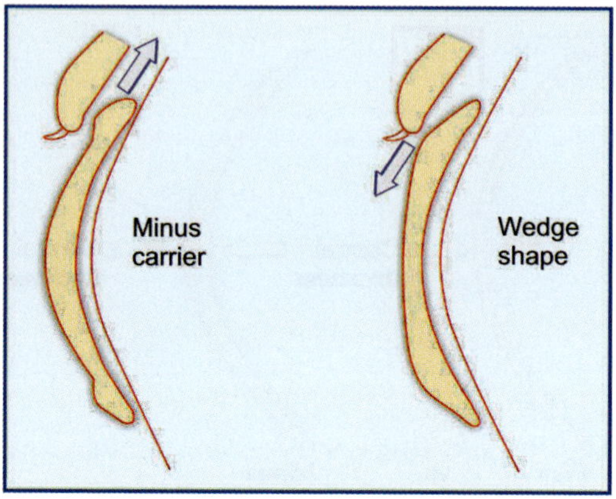

Fig. 3.5: Minus carrier and wedge shape edge and lid interaction

the lens can be made stable by increasing the diameter of the lens by reducing mass by creating a lenticular design or adding minus carrier lenses.

4 Cornea, Oxygen and Contact Lens

In 1946 Goodlaw concluded that oxygen supply was depleted because of contact lenses on the eye and that, oxygen should pass through contact lenses for corneal health.

Subsequently research proved that contact lens induced hypoxia may cause changes in the corneal layers. And now over the years with the origin of newer and better oxygen permeable lenses corneal health is taken care of with contact lenses on the eye.

Let us first understand the basics of **cornea and its oxygen supply.**

When the **eye is open**, the oxygen supply to cornea is through following modes (Fig. 4.1):

1. Posteriorly—by diffusion through aqueous.
2. Radially—through limbal vessels.
3. Anteriorly—by diffusion across the tear film from the atmosphere.

When the **eye is closed**, the supply from atmosphere is cut off and thus remains through:

1. Palpebral conjunctival blood vessels.
2. Limbal route which supplies oxygen to peripheral 1 mm of cornea.
3. Some may enter through the palpebral fissure, if the lids are not tightly closed.

Oxygenation of anterior cornea underneath a contact lens is brought about by diffusion of atmospheric oxygen through the contact lens and the influx of oxygenated tear fluid underneath

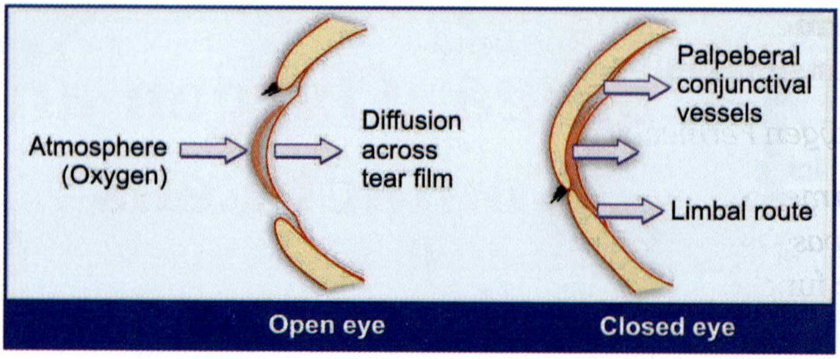

Fig. 4.1: Open eye closed eye

the contact lens as a result of blinking. This tear pump is the only source of oxygen in case of PMMA lenses. However, the tear pump alone is insufficient to provide the adequate amounts of the oxygen required by the cornea.

The **tear pump** supplies about 14 to 20% tear exchange underneath a RGP lens (depends on design also) whereas a soft lens exchanges tears from 1-5% only. The tear pump supplies oxygen and nutrients to the cornea and also remove the waste products like the carbon dioxide, lactic acid and dead epithelia cells (Fig. 4.2).

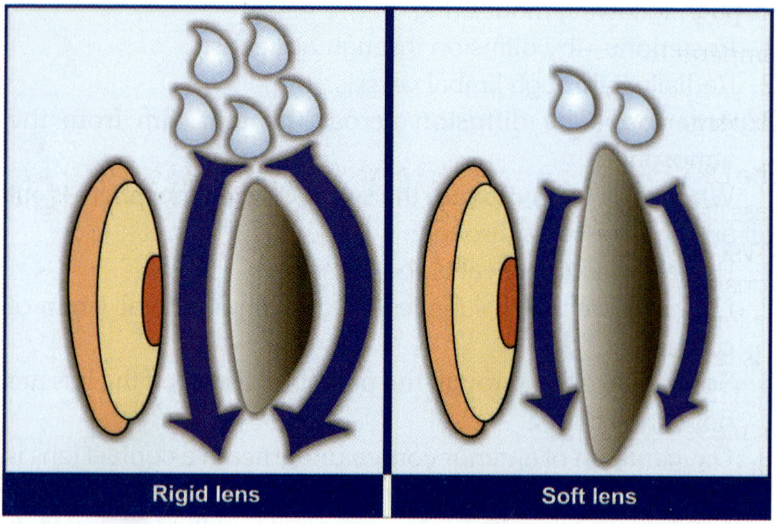

Fig. 4.2: Tear exchange soft vs rigid

Permeability of Materials Dk and Transmissibility of Contact Lenses Dk/L

Oxygen Permeability–Dk

Permeability is the degree to which a substance (oxygen) is able to pass through a membrane or other material. Permeability is the function of the molecular composition of the material.

Though, fixed for each material, yet may depend upon factors such as concentration, temperature, pressure and humidity.

The permeability of a material is denoted as permeability coefficient Dk.

Dk: D is Diffusion Coefficient and k is the Solubility Coefficient

D is the speed with which the gas molecules travel (diffuse) through a material.

And k is defined as how much oxygen can be dissolved in a unit volume of a material at a specified pressure.

A Dk value is expressed in standard units: also called as **Barrer.**

10.9×10^{-11} (cm^2/sec) ml O_2/ml × mm Hg)@ specified temperature.

Oxygen Transmissibility–Dk/L

The Dk value of a material is not how much oxygen will actually pass through a given contact lens. *The actual rate at which oxygen will pass through a lens of given thickness is called oxygen transmissibility.*

It is denoted by Dk/L. Where Dk is oxygen permeability and L is lens thickness in centimeters.

Transmissibility may thus decrease as the lens thickness increases. It also depends upon the design of the contact lens. Dk/L is expressed as **Barrer/cm,** e.g. 10.9×10^{-9} barrer /cm.

Methods for Measuring Dk

Principle of Measuring Technique

The lens material is placed in contact with a polarographic electrode. As the atmospheric oxygen passes through the contact lens material, an electrical current is created proportional to the amount of oxygen passing through it. **Professor Irving Fatt** contributed to introduction of this polorographic technique (Fig. 4.3).

The three methods commonly used are:

1. Uncorrected Fatt or **Original Fatt**—It is the basic technique, which utilizes the above principle.
2. Corrected Fatt or **Modified Fatt** method—This method takes into account the oxygen passage under the lens correcting it for its edges and boundaries. Values obtained are about 25% less than the uncorrected method technique.
3. **Coulometric technique**—This method measures the Dk in more natural conditions like on eye. The basic principle is the same but the measurements are done with the lens surface covered by aqueous (water) layer on both the surfaces. This method is the most common method used in measuring Dk.

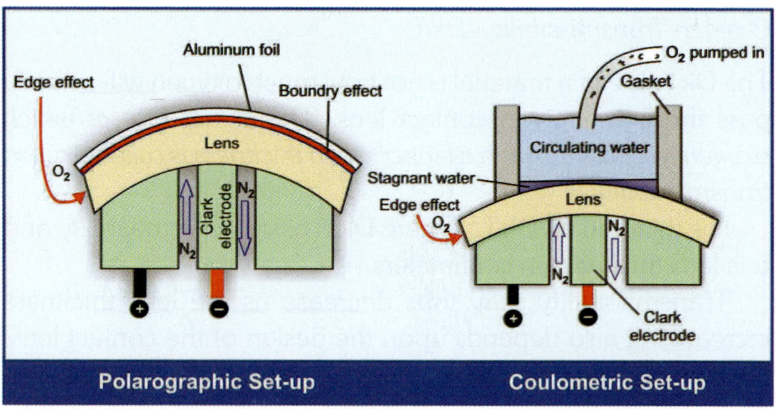

Fig. 4.3: Measurement of Dk

It is important that to compare the Dk of two different materials the method used to measure the Dk should also be specified as comparison can only be true only if the method is same.

The Dk/L of the lenses mentioned by manufacturers, usually is for central thickness measured for –3.0 sphere lens power (as it is midrange minus power) and +3.0 sphere power's central thickness is used for plus powers.

Whereas in actuality the lens is not of uniform thickness, the minus lens is thicker at the periphery and the plus lens is thicker at the center. So sometimes another method is used in measuring Dk /L by taking average thickness of the lens. This is written as **L** avg. This is dependent on the design of the lens and the mathematical calculations are very complex and difficult at times.

Higher Dk vs Lower Dk Material

The material with higher Dk will allow more oxygen to pass through.

Thin vs Thick Lens (Fig. 4.4A)

If the material is same and thickness different, then the thinner lens will allow more oxygen to pass through.

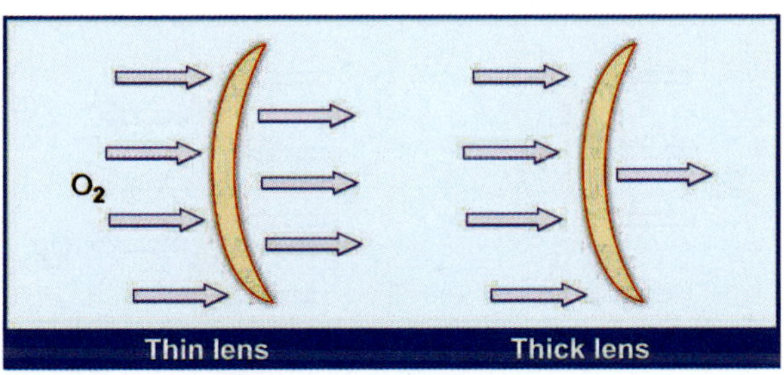

Fig. 4.4A: Dk-thin vs thick lens

Plus Lens vs Minus Lens

The plus lens has a thicker center and thinner periphery. So the transmissibility of oxygen is less in the center. In case of minus powers the periphery is thicker which reduces the transmissibility at the periphery. The hypoxic complications are more likely to happen in the center in plus lenses and in periphery in case of minus lenses.

Dk and Water Content (Fig. 4.4B)

Dk is directly proportional to water content of a material. The higher the water content greater is the Dk.

Unfortunately higher Water content lenses cannot be made thinner as that may lead to rapid dehydration, corneal desiccation and may make the lens more fragile.

It is not necessary that the higher water content lens will have higher transmissibility.

Let us take an example:

Lens A	*Lens B*
Dk = 10×10^{-11}	Dk = 20×10^{-11}
Water content—38%	Water content—76%
Central thickness—	Central thickness—
0.07 mm = 0.007 cm	0.14 mm = 0.014 cm
Dk/L = 10×10^{-11} / 0.007	Dk/L = 20×10^{-11} / 0.014
Dk /L = 14.2×10^{-9}	Dk /L = 14.1×10^{-9}

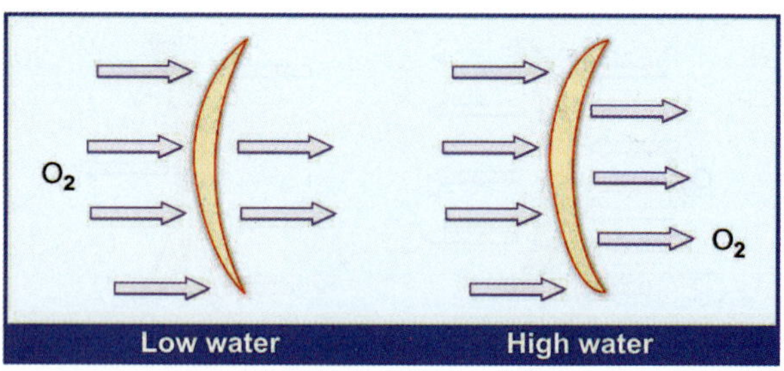

Fig. 4.4B: Dk and water content

Oxygen Flux

It is another physical measure of measuring oxygen transmissibility and permeability in laboratory or *in vitro* technique.

It is defined as the amount of the oxygen that passes through the specified area of the contact lens per unit time, usually specified in minutes or hours. It is expressed in units of $\mu l\ O_2/\ cm^2 \times$ minute.

This can be measured by coulometric technique and *gives more accurate indication of true oxygen transmissibility under a lens.*

Equivalent Oxygen Performance (EOP)

This is an *in vivo technique*, which means it measures the actual oxygen performance of the lens on a living eye.

Principle of this measurement is based on the fact that the cornea is taking oxygen from the atmosphere and this average uptake measures the oxygen transmitted through the lens.

Method of Measuring EOP

A sensor containing a membrane saturated with oxygen is placed onto the corneal surface. As the cornea consumes the oxygen from this sensor the sensor measures the consumption in terms of electric current flowing through it. So, first measure the EOP without the lens and then the EOP with the lens on the eye. Compare to find out the oxygen transmittance through the lens.

Studies have shown that the average rate of oxygen uptake for the cornea is from 3.5 to 7.0 $\mu lO_2/\ cm^2$ per hour.

The atmosphere contains 21% of oxygen by volume or 155 mm Hg of pressure. Thus an ideal contact lens will maintain an EOP of 21%. This means that a lens with 21% EOP is 100 % permeable to oxygen. So in case the EOP value is 10.5 it signifies that the lens is 50% permeable to oxygen.

EOP measures the oxygen permeability *in vivo* conditions compared to the Dk which is *in vitro* condition. Both values cannot be converted into each other.

How much Oxygen Level is Needed for Safe Contact Lens Wear?

When the eye is closed the atmospheric supply of oxygen is cut off and the average oxygen pressure reduces to 55 mm Hg or 6 to 7% which is supplied by the limbal capillaries and the palpebral conjunctiva. Due to this, in a non-lens wearing eye also the cornea also swells to approximately 5-6% during sleep. This reduces immediately on awakening and the cornea tends to deswell to its normal thickness.

There are no significant clinical changes in the cornea if the edema is upto 5%. If the cornea is deprived further signs and symptoms develop.

The effect of hypoxia may be on all layers of the cornea leading to conditions like, infiltrative keratitis, microcysts, neovascularization, corneal exhaustion syndrome and corneal edema.

Studies have been done to calculate the amount of oxygen levels needed with the contact lens on the eye, for safe contact lens wear on the eye.

One of the studies done by Holden and Mertz in 1984 is as follows. These calculations are done by original Fatt method and calculated the corneal swelling in 36 hours.

In daily wear this states that there is zero percent swelling , in case of extended wear it calculates the Dk/L for 4% corneal swelling (which happens in closed eye without lens also).

Safe wear	*Criteria*	*Dk/L*	*EOP*
Safe daily wear	Zero day 1 swelling	$24.1 + -2.7 \times 10^{-9}$	9.9%
Safe extended wear	4% or less corneal swelling	$87.0 + -3.3 \times 10^{-9}$	17.9%

There is also an compromised criteria which suggest the limits of corneal edema to 8% (allowing for the fact the cornea is able to deswell back to normal thickness shortly after eye opening).

Compromised criterion	Zero day 2 residual swelling	$34.3 +-5.2 \times 10^{-9}$	12.1%

5 Slit-lamp Biomicroscopy and Contact Lens

Slit-lamp is an important tool for the assessment of contact lens fitting and the anterior segment of the eye. Gulstrand in 1911 first designed a slit-lamp which was subsequently improved to modern slit-lamp designs.

The slit-lamp biomicrosope consists of 3 parts (Fig. 5.1):

1. The observation system—which includes the microscope to obtain magnification.
2. The illumination system—which illuminates the part to be seen.
3. The mechanical support system—for accurate and convenient positioning of the eye and the instrument.

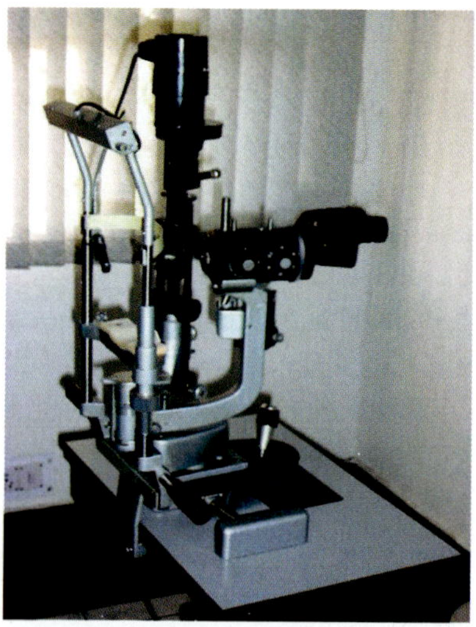

Fig. 5.1: Slit-lamp

SLIT-LAMP ILLUMINATION TECHNIQUES

The ability to detect and observe various anterior segment condition depends upon the observer to correctly adjust and position the illumination system of the slit-lamp.

The illumination techniques can be broadly categorized into 4 main categories:

1. Diffuse
2. Direct
3. Indirect
4. Filtered.

Diffuse Illumination

It is called so because a diffuse filter is placed in the focused light beam of the slit-lamp. This gives an even broad illumination over the entire eye.

To Set Up (Fig. 5.2)

- Angle between slit-lamp and microscope is from 10 to 70 degrees.
- Wide beam.
- Diffusing filter in place.
- Low to medium magnification.

Used to Observe (Fig. 5.3)

- General view and gross screening of the eye, cornea and conjunctiva.
- Contact lens fitting performance.

Direct Illumination

Direct illumination means that the *observing system is focusing directly at the area under illumination.*

It is further classified into following:

1. Optic section
2. Parallelepiped

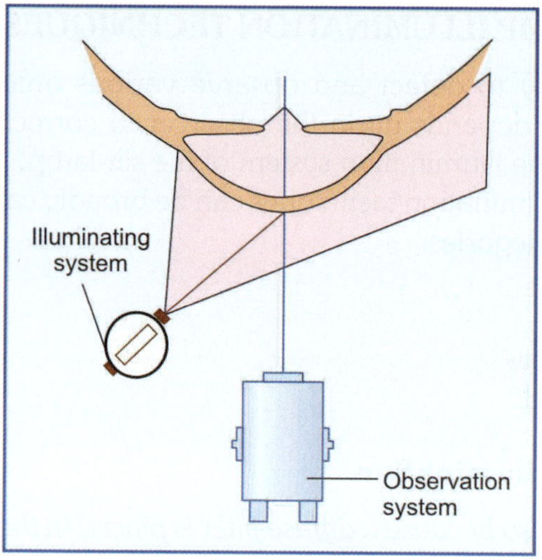

Fig. 5.2: Diffuse illumination set-up

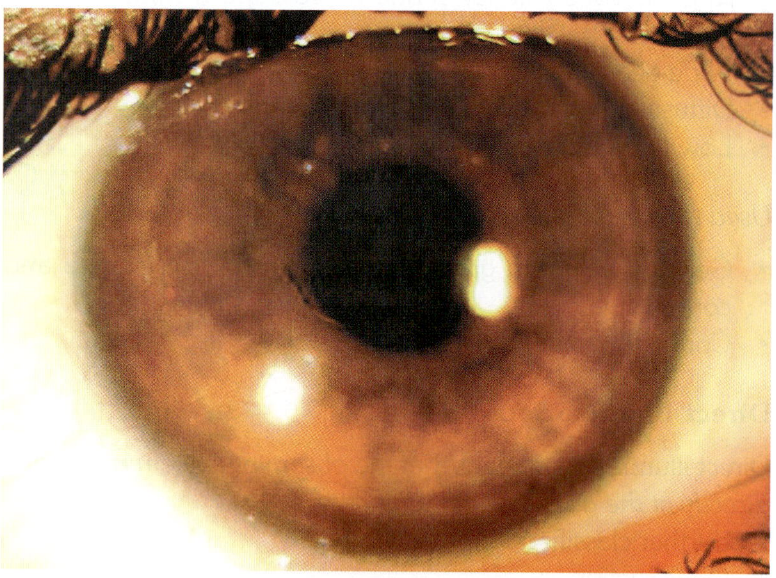

Fig. 5.3: Diffuse illumination

3. Broad beam
4. Conical beam
5. Specular reflection.

Optic Section

This technique utilizes a narrow, focused slit of 0.02 to 0.1 mm to produce a cross-section view especially of the cornea.

To Set Up (Fig. 5.4)

- 30 to 60 degrees angle between observation and illumination system.
- Medium to high illumination.

Used to Observe (Fig. 5.5)

- Variation in corneal curvature.
- Corneal thickness.
- Depth of corneal opacities.
- Foreign body embedded in cornea.

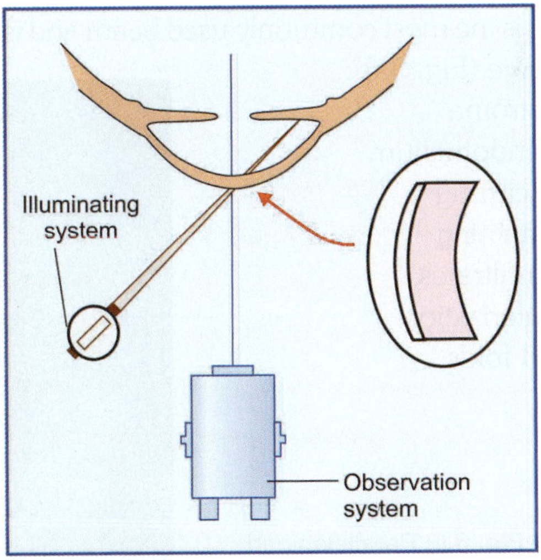

Fig. 5.4: Optic section set-up

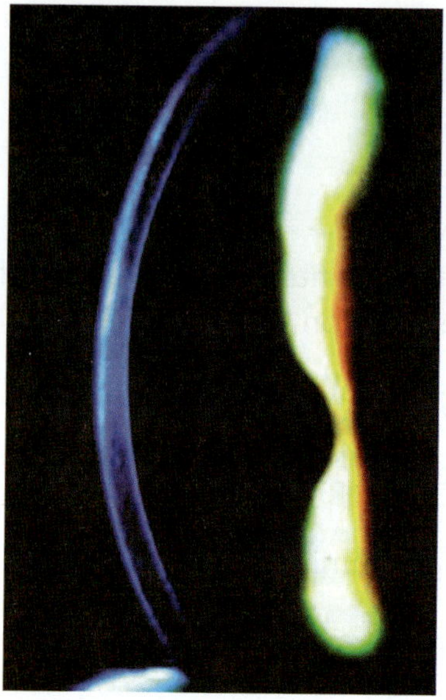

Fig. 5.5: Optic section of cornea

Parallelepiped

This illumination is same as optic section except *that the beam is broader than optic section.* The size of the beam is 0.1 to 0.7 mm. This is the most commonly used beam and is commonly used to observe (Fig. 5.6):

- Corneal stroma
- Corneal endothelium
- Corneal scarring
- Corneal staining
- Corneal infiltrates
- Neovascularization
- Striae and folds.

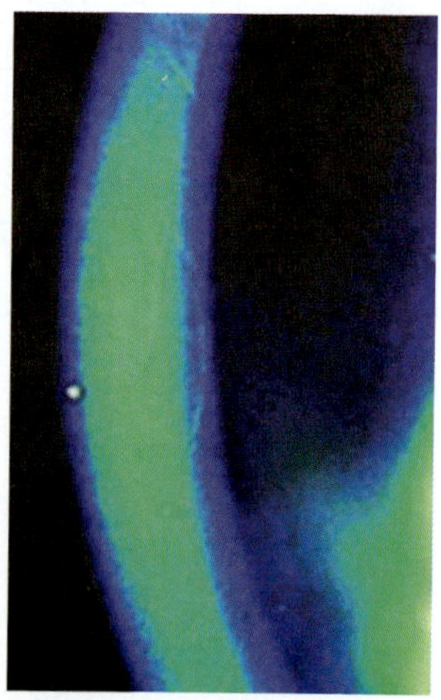

Fig. 5.6: Parallelepiped showing striae in the cornea

Broad Beam Illumination

This is further widening of parallelepiped illumination beam to 1 to 5 mm (Fig. 5.7).

This is used to observe:

- Corneal nerve fibers.
- Debris beneath the contact lens.
- Conjunctival scars (Fig. 5.8).

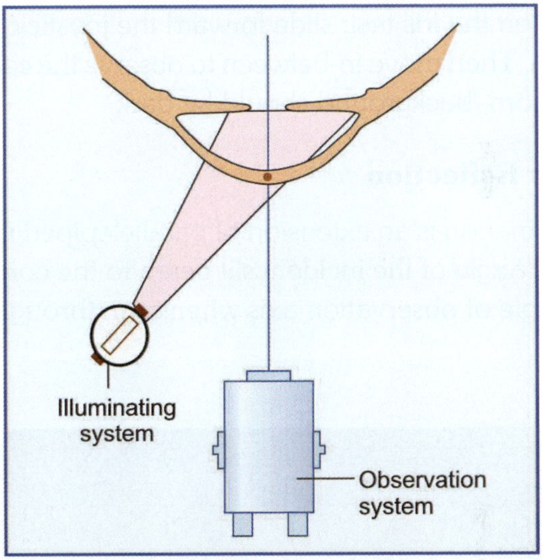

Fig. 5.7: Broad beam set-up

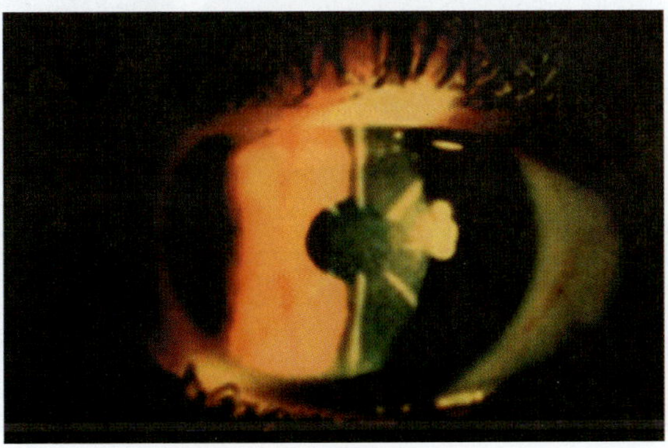

Fig. 5.8: Broad beam

Conical Beam Illumination

This beam is utilized to observe the inflammatory cells or flare in the anterior chamber (Fig. 5.9).

To Set Up

- Same as optic section.
- Reduce the height of the beam to 1 to 2 mm.
- Focus on the iris first; slide forward the joystick to focus the cornea. Then move in-between to observe the cells and flare.
- The room /background should be dark.

Specular Reflection

This illumination is an extension of parallelepiped illumination, where the angle of the incident slit beam to the corneal surface equals angle of observation axis when seen through one of the oculars.

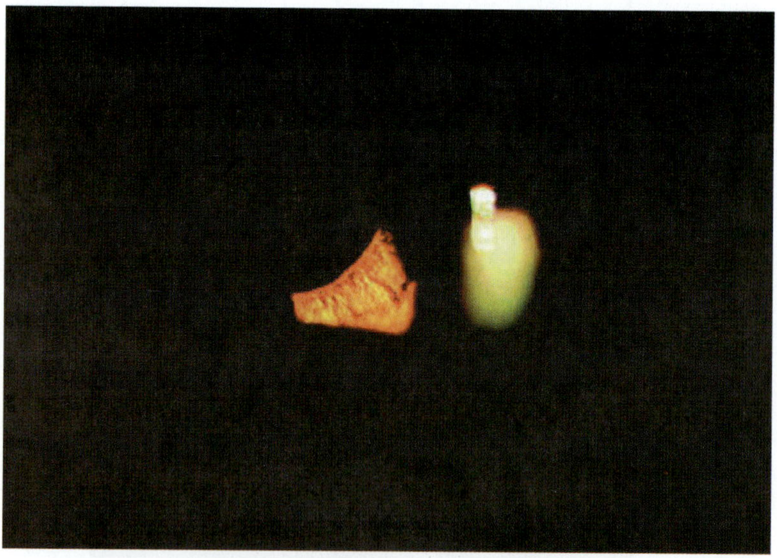

Fig. 5.9: Conical beam to observe anterior chamber

To Set Up (Fig. 5.10)

- 60 degrees angle between illumination and observation system.
- Parallelepiped.
- Move illumination arm until bright reflex is observed. At this point the angle of incidence is equal to angle of reflection.
- See through one oculars.
- Shift magnification to high now.
- Observe the endothelium mosaic in the dull image next to the bright reflex.

Used to Observe

- Endothelial mosaic along with guttae, folds, blebs.
- Tear layer stability and lipid layer.
- Lens front surface wetting.

Indirect Illumination

This refers to any technique where the *focus of the illumination beam does not coincide with the observation system.*

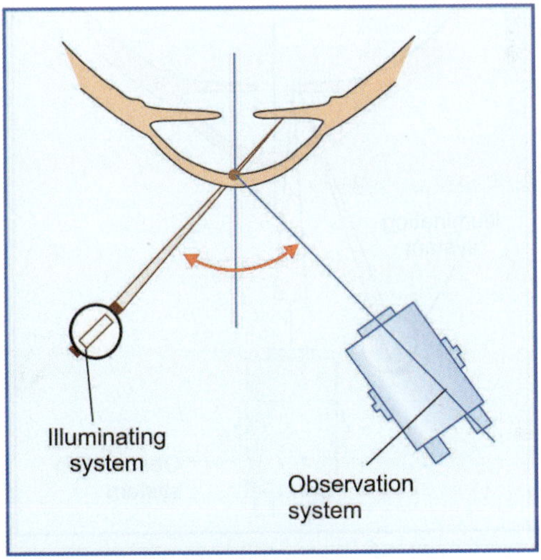

Fig. 5.10: Specular reflection set-up

The two major indirect illuminations are:
- Retroillumination
- Sclerotic scatter.

Retroillumination

This is further of two types:
- Direct
- Indirect

The light is reflected off the iris or fundus while the microscope is focused on the cornea.

To Set Up

- Offset the slit-beam.
- Create a parallelepiped beam.
- Illuminate the area behind the corneal area to be seen.
- Observe the cornea in the reflected light.
- Direct—See the corneal just in front of the illuminated area (Fig. 5.11).

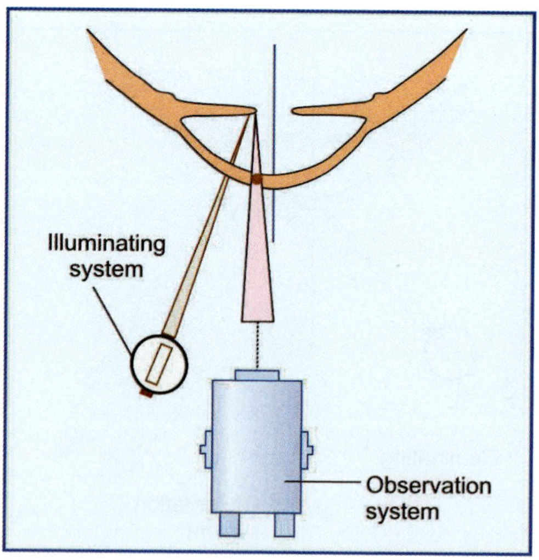

Fig. 5.11: Direct retroillumination set-up

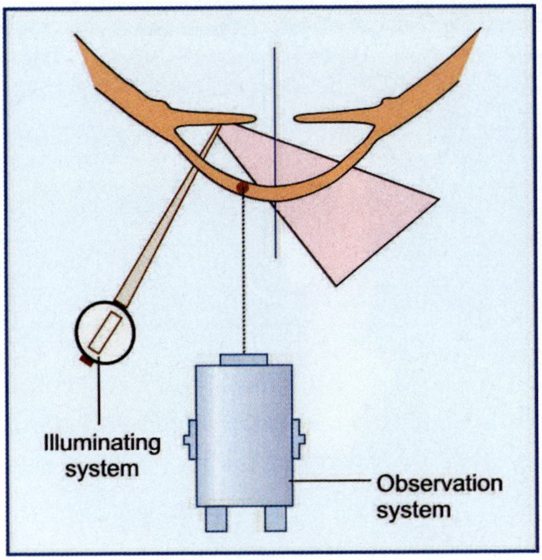

Fig. 5.12: Indirect retroillumination set-up

- Indirect—See the corneal area adjacent to the illuminated area (Fig. 5.12).

Used to Observe (Figs 5.13 and 5.14)

- Contact lens front and back surface deposits.
- Neovascularization, edema.
- Microcysts.
- Infiltrates.

Sclerotic Scatter

This is a type of indirect illumination.

To Set Up (Fig. 5.15)

- Utilizes a parallelepiped technique.
- Focus the beam on the nasal or temporal limbus.
- Light from the slit is totally internally reflected and the cornea glows.
- Observe the cornea against the bright glow.

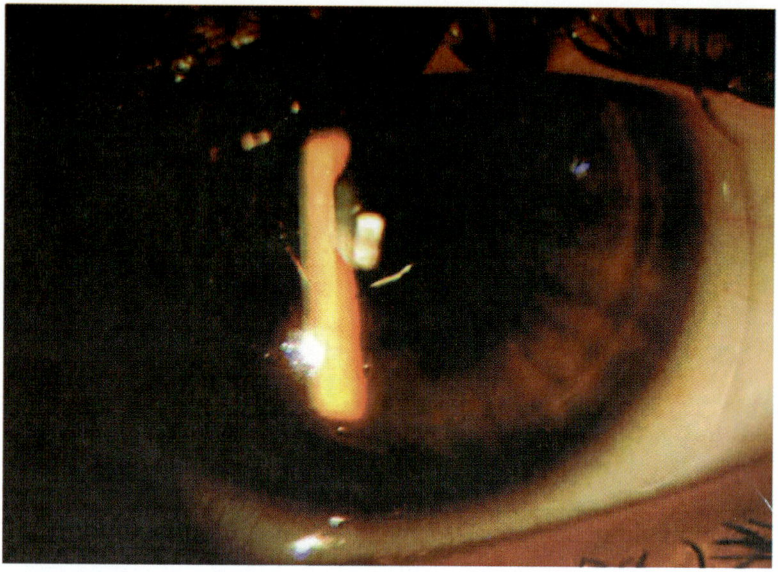

Fig. 5.13: A torn lens seen by direct retroillumination

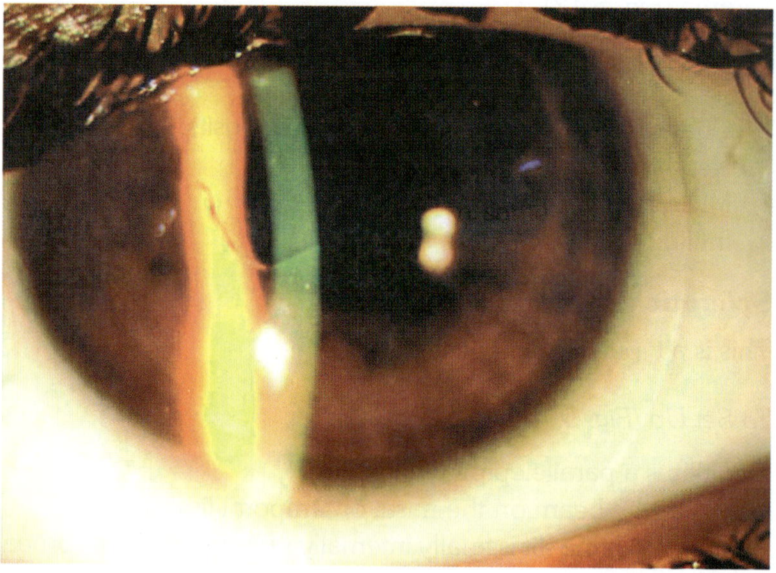

Fig. 5.14: The torn lens seen by indirect retroillumination

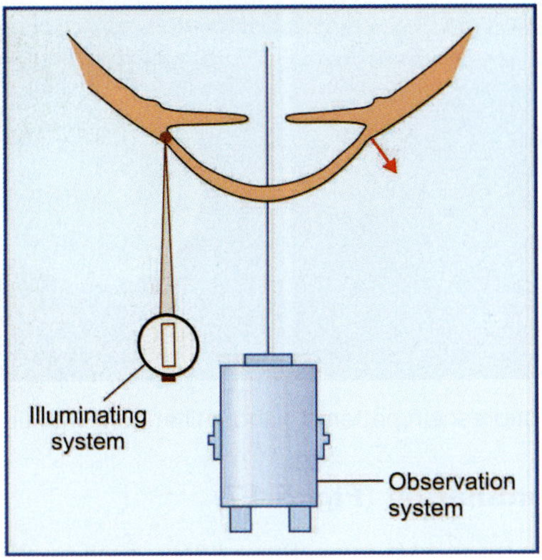

Fig. 5.15: Sclerotic scatter set-up

Used to Observe (Fig. 5.16)

- Central corneal clouding.
- Corneal scars.
- Foreign body/deposits.

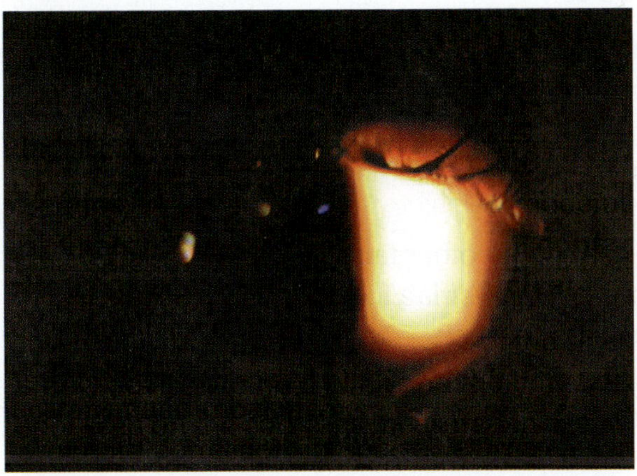

Fig. 5.16: Sclerotic scatter

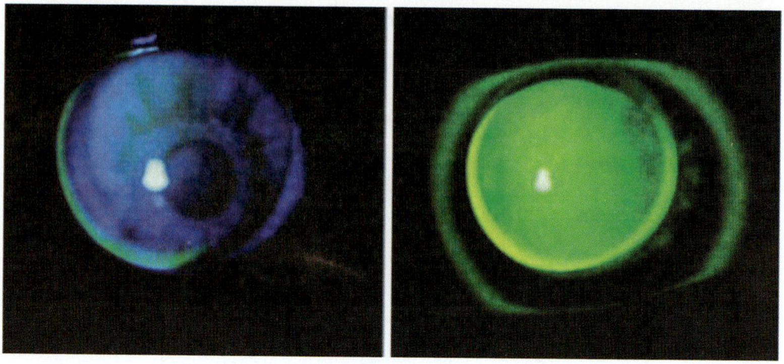

Fig. 5.17: Fluorescein patterns without filter (left) with filter (right)

Filtered Illumination (Fig. 5.17)

Cobalt blue light and Wratten filter #12 – (yellow filter) is used to observe the corneal staining patterns and rigid gas permeable lens fitting relationship on the eye. This is frequently used illumination where the fluorescein dye and the filter is used to highlight the eye condition and the fitting. The yellow filter is an added attachment which when used with cobalt blue light enhances the contrast further and makes the observation easier.

Abnormalities

Checklist to be seen by slit-lamp during contact lens examination:

1. Blepharitis
2. Cornel infiltrates
3. Iritis
4. Ulcer
5. Papillae or any other tarsal conjunctival abnormalities
6. Corneal edema/striae/folds
7. Neovascularization
8. Corneal staining
9. Microcysts
10. Endothelial status.

6 Keratometry and Corneal Topography

The most common method of measurement of corneal curvature in contact lens practice is the keratometry, although recently there has been increasing use of videokeratoscopy or topography.

LET US REVISE

Corneal Diameter

- HVID = 10 to 14 mm (average : 11.7 mm) and
- VVID average = 10.6 mm
- The average central radius of curvature is 7.8 mm at the central cap region.
- In early life, cornea is found to be having WTR (with the rule) astigmatism.
- Cornea is aspheric. (Asphericity – It is the measure of the deviation of the peripheral surface curvature from the apical curvature). To measure asphericity following terms are used: Eccentricity = e and shape factor = p.

Eccentricity Value of the Human Cornea

- The human cornea is an ellipsoid.
- Eccentricity value that have been given are: Range: 4.41 – 0.58 (Average: 0.47).

Instruments Used to Study the Corneal Topography

- Placido's disk (Fig. 6.1)

- Photokeratoscope (Fig. 6.2)
- Keratometer (Fig. 6.3)
- VKG (videokeratograph)
- ORB-scan.

Ophthalmometer

Ophthalmometer is the instrument used to measure the radius of anterior corneal surface. Keratometer is the trade name for the Baush and Lomb Ophthalmometer.

Types of Keratometers

- Baush and Lomb keratometer—One position keratometer.
- Javal and Schiotz keratometer—Two position keratometer.

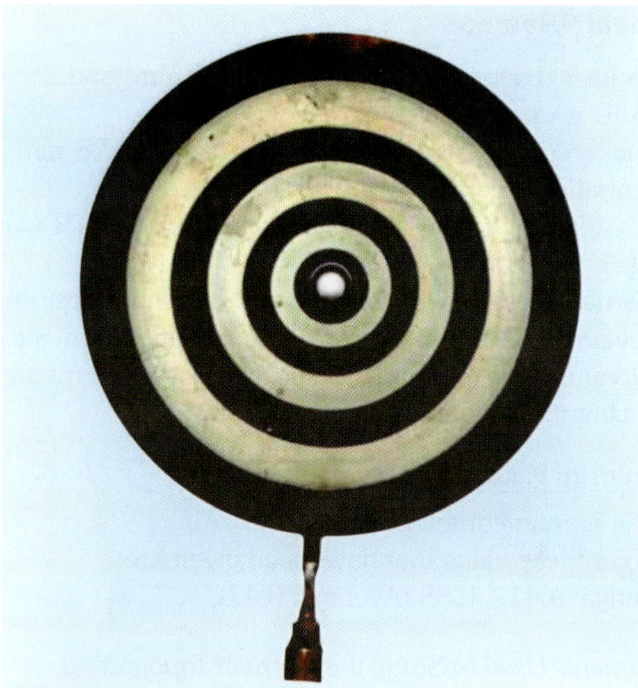

Fig. 6.1: Placido's disk

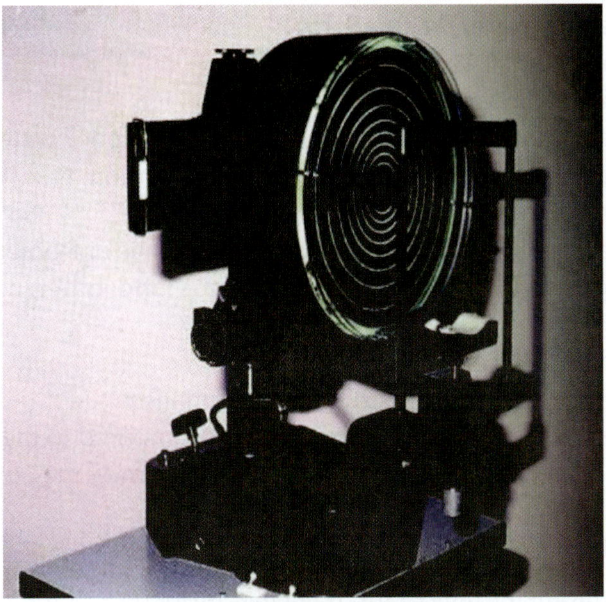

Fig. 6.2: Photokeratoscope

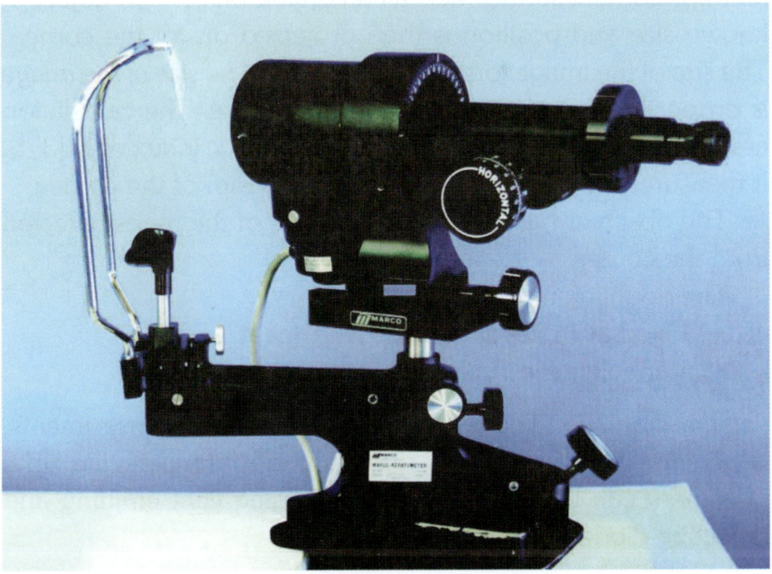

Fig. 6.3: Keratometer

The keratometer is used for:

- Contact lens base curve selection.
- Detect RGP lens flexure.
- Detect contact lens deposits, irregularities, poor wetting.
- Detect and monitor corneal surface distortion.
- Estimate refractive astigmatism.
- Differentially diagnose axial versus refractive anisometropia.
- Diagnose and monitor keratoconus and other corneal disease.
- Calculate IOL power.
- Monitor intra and postsurgical astigmatism.

Keratometer has following limitation compared to the topography that, it can measure only central 3 mm of the cornea.

Principle

The keratometer utilizes the reflective properties of the cornea to measure the radius of curvature of the anterior cornea. The anterior corneal surface acts as a convex mirror. An object of known size and position is then projected on tot the cornea. The size of the image formed is measured. *The size of the image is proportional to the radius of the curvature.* The calculation assumes the cornea to be sphere and refractive index of 1.3375. It measures the curvature in the central 3 mm of the cornea.

The observer has to align the images of the mires reflected from the cornea.

The doubling may be:

- Fixed as in Javal Schoitz instrument
- Variable as in Baush and Lomb Keratometer.

Autokeratometer: These are usually two position instruments, which use servometers to drive the doubling device until alignment can be assessed optically, using light emitting and detecting diodes.

Overview of Steps in Taking Measurements— (Baush and Lomb Keratometer)

1. Adjust eye pieces according to your eye.
2. Position the patient comfortable with the chin and the head resting properly and firmly against the chinrest and the head rest.
3. Adjust the height of the face, such that the lateral canthus coincides with the line on outer rim.
4. Occlude the non examining eye. Ask the patient to fix with the eye to be examined to the centre of the mires.
5. Locate the mire image on the cornea from the outside first.
6. Focus the center circle of the mire image while keeping the black cross in its center (Figs 6.4 and 6.5).
7. Coincide the axis line of the plus sign mire.
8. Coincide, the two minus signs and the two plus signs.
9. If the readings fall out of the keratometer range (36.0 D to 52.0 D) use an auxiliary lens in front of the objective to increase the range. Refer to the nomograms to get the final reading corresponding to the one read with the auxillary lens.
   - Attach - +1.25 Ds—for readings above 52.0 D—Add approximately 8.0 to the reading read on the drum.

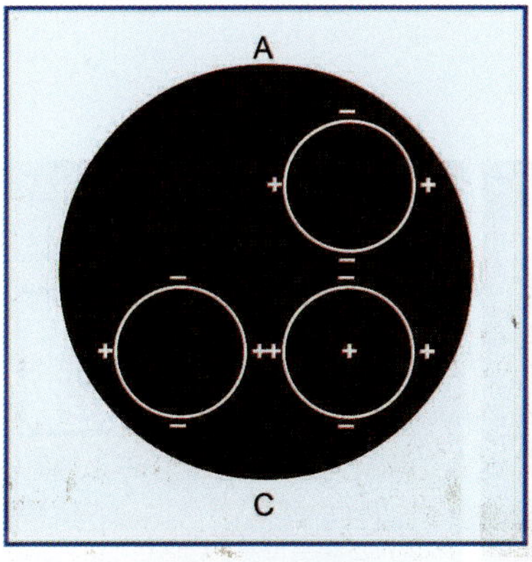

Fig. 6.4: Focused mires

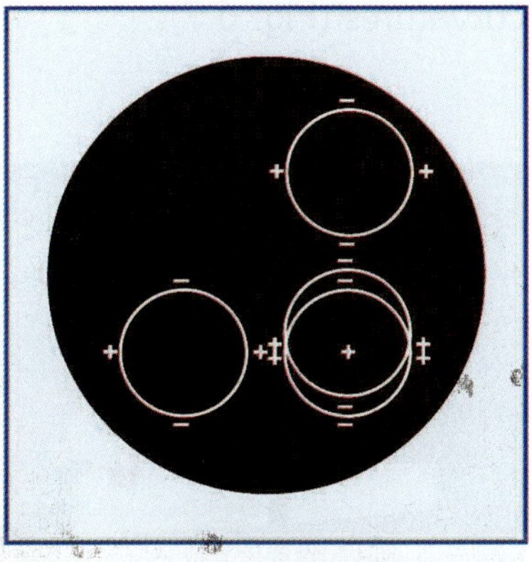

Fig. 6.5: Keratometer mires defocused

- Attach -1.25 Ds—for readings below 36.0 D—Subtract 6.0 D from the reading now read on the drum.

CORNEAL TOPOGRAPHY

Computer generated 3-dimensional corneal map

Topography is defined as the science of describing or representing the feature of a particular place in detail. Corneal topography measures the shape and the curvature of the anterior corneal surface (Fig. 6.6).

The videokeratoscope has made it possible to computer analyze the corneal curvature and shape. It uses 15 to 32 concentric rings as illuminated target and radius of curvature is presented as color code. The instrument has given the Practitioner the means of looking at the corneal contour with far more accuracy now.

Computerized Video Keratography (VKG)

In 1988, Klyce started with the color corneal maps.

The warm colors—red and orange are used to represent relatively higher power that is steeper curvature and green and yellow colors are associated with normal cornea. Cool colors hues of blue—used to represent relatively lower powers, i.e. flatter curvatures (Fig. 6.7).

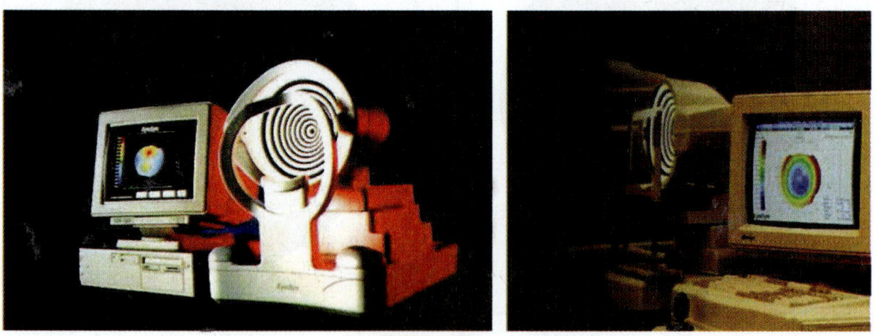

Fig. 6.6. Corneal topographers

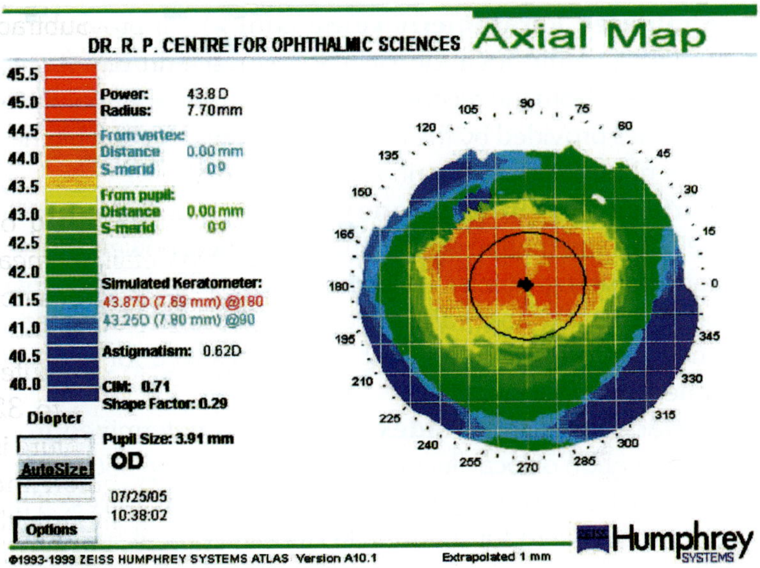

Fig. 6.7: A topographer print

Uses of VKG

- To study normal topography.
- To help explain uncorrected acuity.
- In research instruments for measuring detailed topography and image data analysis.
- To study the effect of disease.
- To monitor progressive changes, especially in keratoconus.
- In Pre and postsurgical comparison.
- In Penetrating keratoplasty surgery.
- To study the effect of contact lenses. Monitor changes caused by different CL wear modalities.
- Manage corneal changes in orthokeratology.

Interpretation of Corneal Topography

The following readings are compared to define the corneal shape and asymmetry:

- Elevation maps.

- **Simulated keratometry value (sim k)**—it provides the power and the location of the steepest and the flattest meridians from the reconstructed corneal surface analogous to values provided by the keratometer. This can be obtained from photokeratoscope ring numbers 7,8,9.
- **Surface asymmetry index (SAI)**—it is the centrally weighted summation of differences in corneal power between corresponding points. These points are 180 degrees apart on 128 equally spaced meridians that cross the four central photokeratoscope mires. SAI approaches zero for perfectly spherical surfaces.
- **Surface regularity index (SRI)**—it is determined from a summation of local fluctuations in power along 256 equally spaced hemi-meridians on the 10 central mires. This approaches zero for a normally smooth corneal surface.

As a contact lens practitioner it forms a very useful tool in fitting abnormal corneas (Fig. 6.8).

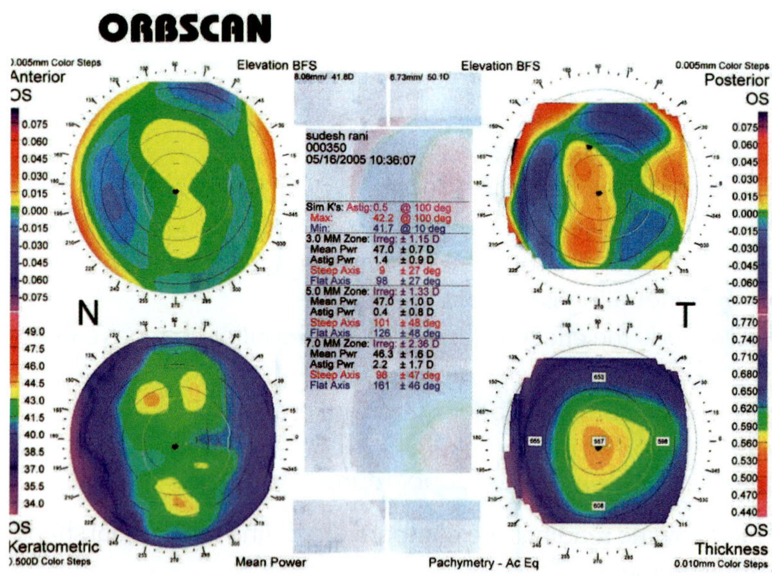

Fig. 6.8: A topographer print

It is an indispensable tool for finding a starting point for unusual corneas in contact lens fitting. Most of these systems are equipped with the option of purchasing a contact lens fitting program.

Contact Lens Fitting Assisted with Topographer

Once you enter the patient's refractive error into the fitting program, the instrument can calculate the design. The computer will generate a listing of the base curve, diameter, optic zone diameter, peripheral curves, etc. These programs may also provide guidelines related to the fitting and display a fluorescein pattern simulation, which illustrates the expected fitting relationship of the lens to the cornea.

7 Contact Lens Materials

The history of the contact lens clearly shows the development of newer and newer materials that satisfied the needs of the patient, practitioner and the manufacturer. All present day sophisticated researches approach towards improving the lens materials to a one that can be physiologically ideal for the eye and can be worn for continuously. We still look forward to that ideal lens material.

An **ideal contact lens material** is the one, which would meet the following conditions:

- It provides sufficient oxygen to the cornea to meet its requirements.
- Is optically transparent.
- Has stable dimensions.
- Has good wettability when on the eye.
- It requires minimum patient care and maintenance.
- It resists spoliation.
- Is easily machinable or easy to manufacture.

Physical Properties of the Lens

1. *Wettability*—It is the ability of the tears to form a complete film over the lens surface.
2. *Flexibility*—The, more the lens is rigid the less it will bend when placed over the cornea. A highly flexible material will contour to the cornea.
3. *Optical quality*—The lens should be optically homogenous and transparent with minimum transmission loss.

4. *Biocompatibility*—The lens should not induce any inflammatory or immunological responses and should be inert.
5. *Manufacturing ease*—The process of lens manufacturing should be easy and cost effective.
6. *Stable parameters*—Lens material should be dimensionally stable and be easily polished. The hydrogels should have stable hydration parameters.

Contact lenses are made of plastics, which are synthetic or semisynthetic macromolecular materials called **polymers**.

Chemical Composition of Contact Lens Polymers

Polymers are made by condensation or addition of monomers. When two or more kinds of monomers are combined by polymerization the result is a copolymer. Monomers are combined in random, alternating or chain fashion. The arrangement of monomers effects the properties of the copolymers. These properties also depend upon the method of polymerization.

Thermoplastic polymers: If the contact lens polymer can be melt under heat they are thermoplastic. These can be moulded.

Thermoset plastic: A thermoset plastic does not melt or dissolve.

Monomers can be polymerized to form contact lens rods from which blanks are cut. A lens can be lathed from these blanks.

Spin casting of contact lens is done by polymerizing the material in rotating open moulds. Cast moulding is done by polymerizing the material in closed moulds. Moulding process can be only done to thermoplastic materials.

Classification of Contact Lens Materials (Flow Chart 7.1)

Rigid (Hard) Lenses

Poly (Methyl Methacrylate) PMMA is the backbone of all Rigid lens materials. It was the first rigid lens material which was patented in 1934. It is a thermoplastic material with following properties:

1. Excellent biocompatibility
2. Good optical properties
3. Does not scratch so easily
4. Good manufacturing properties.

Major Drawback

Even though PMMA is an excellent contact lens materials as far as physical properties are concerned, It has a major drawback, that it has extremely low oxygen permeability. This hindered with the corneal physiology and has ultimately made PMMA material an obsolete for use. It produced corneal exhaustion on prolonged use.

The better understanding of the cornea contact lens and oxygen stimulated the search of new materials with higher oxygen permeability (Fig. 7.1).

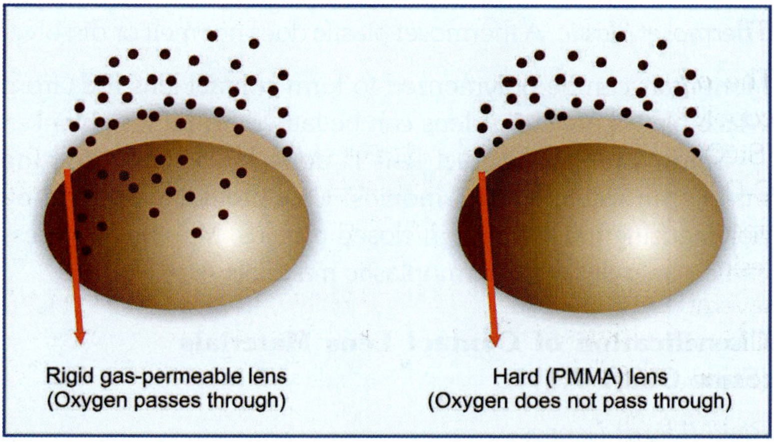

Fig. 7.1: Oxygen permeable rigid contact lens vs PMMA lens

PMMA (Polymethyl methacrylate)

— 1934
— Good optics
— Easy to manufacture
— Very stable
— Easily wettable
— Almost zero O_2.

OXYGEN PERMEABLE RGP MATERIALS

Cellulose Acetate Butyrate

CAB is an early contact lens material derived from an natural polysaccharide—cellulose. It usually contains about 13% acetyl groups, 37% butyryl groups and 1 to 2% free hydroxyl groups. It is an thermoplastic which had relatively higher oxygen permeability compared to PMMA. It can absorb 2% of moisture, which in turn may lead to warping and distortion. It has a low Dk in the range of 4-8 and was difficult to manufacture by lathing technique. This material is also not compatible with benzalkonium chloride an common preservative in CL solutions.

Siloxane Methacrylate

The oxygen permeability of rigid lenses was improved by copolymerization of methyl methacrylate with certain Siloxane (Si–O-Si), alkyl (-CH_2-CH_2- CH_2-) and methacrylate (CH_2= C-COO-) monomers. The permeability of this polymer depends upon the distribution of Siloxane bonds. Compared to silicone resins these have a backbone of carbon to carbon linkages with several branches of Siloxane bonds. Also these do not contain silicone so are not called silicon methacrylates. Several other compounds are added to improve its rigidity and wettability.

This is the most successful rigid gas-permeable material even today, which was introduced in 1970. The Dk values of 12 to 60 are achievable in this group. These lenses had a negative charge due to which they are more deposit prone. Their surface also scratches easily and may cause flexure problems if made thinner than the critical thickness.

Some examples of Siloxane acrylate materials are, Boston II, IV, Ablerta II, III, Menicon O_2, and Polycon II.

Fluoro-Siloxane-methacrylates

These materials were derived from Siloxanelalkyl methacrylate but in addition contain some fluorinated monomers. The addition of fluorine improved the oxygen permeability of Siloxane methacrylates further. The Dk achieved ranges from 40 to 100 or more which makes it possible for extended wear also. The surface of these materials has less charge than the Siloxane acrylates but may be more prone to deposits and flexure. Some examples of such material lenses are Fluorperm, Fluorex, Quantum II, Alberta and Equalens.

Alkyl Styrene Copolymers—Butyl Styrene

These materials are low density materials which have better oxygen permeability due to their looseness in the range of 25, still not competitive. Alkyl styrene are made from copolymers with hydrophilic monomers such as vinyl pyrolindine or hydroxymethyl methacrylate. The refractive index of t- butyl styrene was high and the specific gravity low which made the lens thin as well as light especially for high powers. Yet this material is not so much in commercial use.

Rigid gas permeable—RGP

- RGP—combine the desirable qualities of PMMA with increase oxygen permeability.
- Early CAB, Siloxane acrylates T-butyl styrene.

FLEXIBLE FLUOROPOLYMER LENS—PERFLUOROETHERS

Fluorocompounds have relatively high oxygen permeability low refractive index and high density. Perfluoroether compounds have fluorine, carbon, hydrogen and oxygen which are combined with other copolymers like methyl methacrylate/vinyl pyrolidone to obtain material of high oxygen permeability Dk of more than 90. These are flexible materials so are manufactured by moulding procedure and is expensive Example of such lens material is advent.

ELASTOMERIC LENSES

Silicone Rubber

The silicone rubbers are organic—inorganic polymers with a backbone of silicone and oxygen linkages. However, the high oxygen permeability of silicone rubbers have made them very attractive for contact lens use, their hydrophobicity has been a strong deterrent. The surface of this hydrophobic material is made hydrophilic by chemical treatment or coatings. The drawback about these was that the coatings were thin and could rub off making the lens again hydrophobic. Another drawback about this excellent oxygen permeable material was that it is lipophilic, absorbing the lipids present in the tear film.

Acrylic Rubber

Acrylic rubber lenses are made of polymers that have carbon to carbon backbone similar to rigid lenses but have acrylic rather than methacrylic monomers in the polymer. The polymer ultimately results into a soft and rubbery material rather than a rigid one. The finished lenses are also called PBAPMA (polybutyl acylate-cobutyl methacrylate) lenses. They have high oxygen permeability and are also hydrophobic like silicone rubbers.

SOFT CONTACT LENSES—HYDROGELS

The original hydrogel contact lens are made of poly (2-hydroxyethyl methacrylate) (PHEMA). This material was patented in 1955 by O Wichterle and D Lim of Czechoslovakia. The HEMA chains are cross linked by an ethylene glycol dimethacrylate bridge. The hydrophilic nature is because of cross linked polymers with carbon to carbon backbone, to which are attached hydrophilic groups. The dry state is called Xerogel. When a xerogel is placed in aqueous environment it swells. The swelling depends upon the character of the polymer and the environment such as pH temperature, etc. There can be some fluctuations in the parameters when on eye.

PHEMA is still the basic lens material in use as the soft lens material:

Some of the physical properties needed in this lens material are:

1. **Water content:** The water content of the soft material ranges from 38 to 80%. Less than 40 percent are called low water content, 40 to 55% are called mid water content and > 55% are called high water content lenses. The higher the water content greater is the oxygen permeability. The low water content lenses have Dk in the range of 5 to 8. The mid water content lenses have Dk in the range of 7 to 19 and high water content lenses have Dk in the range of 18 to 28.

   Low water content lenses have the advantage of being stable, easier to handle, easier to manufacture, more wettable but have a major drawback of having low oxygen permeability. *High water content lenses* on the other hand have higher oxygen permeability but are less stable, fragile, more deposit prone, difficult to manufacture, less dimension stability and thicker due to their lower refractive index.
2. **Elasticity:** The soft lens material has to be elastic so that it can survive the repeated stress of insertion and removal. It should recover its shape very rapidly after stress.
3. **Ionicity:** The soft lens material can be classified into two groups based on ionicity—Ionic or nonionic.

   The ionic material contains a net negative charge on the surface and the nonionic have no net surface charge. The ionic materials are more prone to deposits due to the net surface charge and have better wettability than nonionic lens materials. Their water content may show variation with the changing pH. On the other hand the nonionic lens materials are less deposit prone and may be less wettable also.

The most common compounds added to HEMA to make new generation hydrogels which are:

- PVP—polyvinylpyrrolidone
- MA—methacrylic acid
- MMA—methyl methacrylate
- GMA—glyceryl methacrylate
- DAA—diacetone acrylamide
- PVA—polyvinyl alcohol.

Several compounds are added to hydrogels to improve its properties like wettability, water content, oxygen permeability or Ionicity.

Generic names of hydrogels have a suffix—filcon.

FDA CLASSIFICATION GROUPS

In 1986 US food and drug administration classified hydrogel contact lenses into 4 groups.

Low water—38-50% water content	*High water—51-80%*
Group I—Nonionic low water content	Group II—Nonionic high water content
Group III—Ionic low water content	*Group IV—Ionic high water content*

Soft lens—hydrophilic—water lowring hydrogels

- PHEMA
- O Wichterle and D Lim
- A polar OH group to which water lipole binds
- 38% water content
- Are soft and pliable
- Large lens diameters
- New generation—soft materials—Improved PHEMA, combination of other polymers 2-3

Soft materials and Dk—depends on

- Water content if higher increases Dk
- Material chemistry
- If pH is acidic it reduces water content
- Hypertonicity reduces water content.

Lenses with Rigid Gas Permeable Optics and Soft Hydrophilic Periphery—Hybrid Lenses

The idea of these mixed lenses came in 1970s when hydrogels were getting popular because of their comfort, but were unable to correct vision as good as in rigid lenses. So a rigid center and soft hydrophilic skirt reached the commercial use. This also came in the name of Saturn lenses.

The New Generation Lens Material

They are the silicone hydrogels with very high Dk and used as continuous wear.

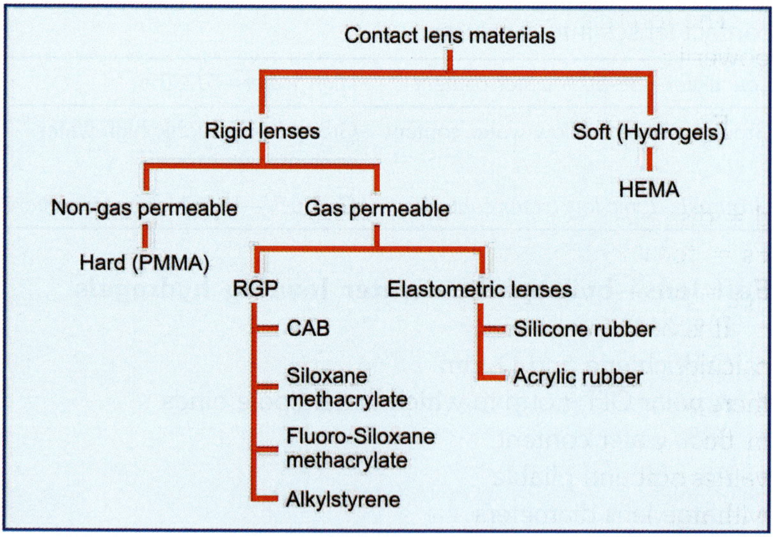

Flow chart 7.1: Showing classifications of contact lens materials

8 Optics of Contact Lens

In this chapter the various optical properties of the contact lens associated with the contact lens fitting and its usage will be briefed.

The contact lens is on the eye and coincides with the corneal plane, so the compensation to the back vertex power of the spectacle power has to be made.

Correction for Vertex Distance

Back vertex power is the distance of the second principal focus from the back vertex of the lens.

The formula used to calculate the contact lens equivalent power is:

$$F_{CL} = \frac{Fs}{(1 - dFs)}$$

d = distance form back vertex of spectacle lens to cornea
Fs = focal length at the spectacle plane
F_{CL} = focal length at the corneal plane.

It is not essential to calculate the back vertex power while calculating lens powers. Usually a correction table should be there with all practitioners as ready reference. The powers stated in this table begin from + /– 4.0 Diopters as below this the values of spectacle and contact lens powers are practically same with not a significant variation.

As a Rule

Minus power—is less in contact lenses compared to spectacles.
Plus power—is higher in contact lenses compared to spectacles.

Spectacle versus Contact Lens Image Size / Magnification

Image size in an optical system is inversely proportional to power of the lens.

In Case of Plus Powers

The image size with contact lenses is smaller than with spectacles. Thus leads to minification.

In Case of Minus Powers

The image size is larger with contact lenses than with spectacles. Thus leads to magnification.

This is a desirable advantage with contact lenses compared to spectacles, more so in case of anisometropes.

Contact lens magnification = 1 – d Fsp

where d = vertex distance
Fsp = focal length of spectacle

When the relative spectacle magnifications are calculated, it has been studied that, In case of axial anisometropes the image size when compared are approximately equal with spectacles. Based on this, theoretically axial anisometropes can be corrected better with spectacles and it is better to correct refractive anisometropes with contact lenses.

Accommodation and Convergence

A Hyperope

A hyperope wearing contact lenses will accommodate less than with spectacles.

A Myope

A Myope wearing contact lens will accommodate more than compared to spectacles.

This may give an advantage of controlling accommodative squint in case of a hyperopes with contact lenses better than the spectacles.

Also a myope whose accommodative demand has increased with lenses when switched from spectacles may cause problems when presbyopia sets in, where it may precipitate early with contact lenses. This means that in case of hyperopes the situation will be better for hyperopic presbyopes.

Convergence

When wearing spectacles the myopic lens behaves as a base in prism so the eye converges less. With contact lenses the myope has to converge more and the hyperope has to converge less.

The Tear Lens (Fig. 8.1)

Between the contact lens and the cornea forms a thin layer of tear film.

This tear film is very thin in case of soft lenses, which drape around the cornea.

Whereas, in rigid lenses this tear layer formed, will depend upon the fitting relationship of the lens and the cornea. *In case of steep fitting the tear lens is a positive lens and in case of flat fitting rigid lens it is a negative lens.*

If the lens is decentered this tear lens will induce a prismatic effect (Fig. 8.2).

If the rigid contact lens is steeper by 0.05 mm or 0.25 diopter A tear lens of = 0.25 Diopters approximately will be formed by this lens. That means that the tear lens will be approximately positive or negative by same amount as much it is steeper or flatter by.

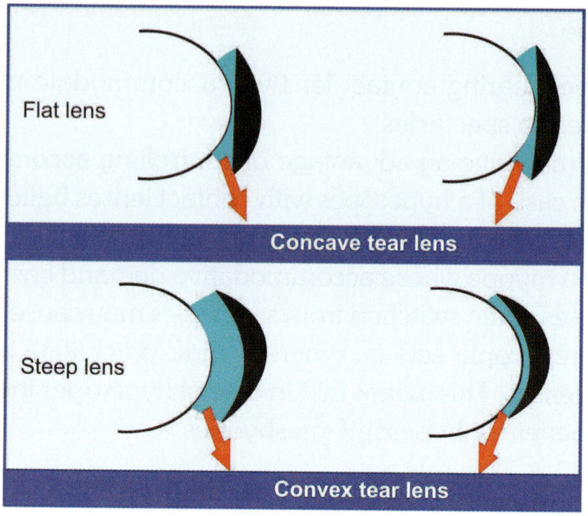

Fig. 8.1: The tear lens

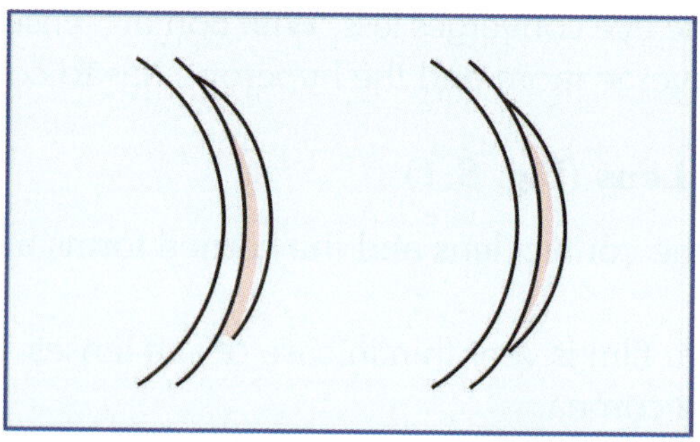

Fig. 8.2: Prismatic effect of tear lens

And the rule is: *0.05 mm Steeper or Flatter will create a tear lens of 0.25 Diopters approx.*

Neutralization of Astigmatism with Rigid Lenses

There is a significant reduction of astigmatic error with spherical rigid lenses. This is based on the assumption that the refractive index of the cornea and the tear is almost same.

In case of spherical rigid lens the tear layer forms a lens between the contact lens and the cornea. This tear layer neutralizes the astigmatism.

About 90% of the astigmatism is neutralized, by the fluid lens, between the cornea and the back surface of the spherical RGP lens. Spherical rigid lenses thus can easily neutralize upto 3 Diopters, of astigmatism.

Field of Vision: Spectacle Compared with Contact Lens

All lenses move with the eye and, hence, the field of vision is better with them when compared to spectacle lenses. Higher the spectacle power greater is the field restriction. So the lenses have a definite advantage over the spectacles by reducing the limitations in the field of view and eliminating the rim interference.

Aberrations Spectacles versus Contact Lenses

As the contact lenses move with the eye the aberrations produced by spectacle lenses are reduced to minimum or eliminated. The chromatic aberration is also very low because the refractive index of the contact lenses is low.

Power of the Contact Lens

The power of the contact lens will depend on two factors

1. Back vertex power.
2. Tear lens power formed between the cornea and the contact lens.

In case of soft lenses the lens is assumed to conform with the cornea so the tear lens is assumed to have zero power. So the CL power is equal to the back vertex power.

In case of rigid lenses the tear lens plays a major role and the final power is equal to BVP + tear lens power.

Rule of Thumb

If the lens is steeper by 0.05 mm, –0.25 D of power should be added to the contact lens or else if it is flatter by 0.50 mm, +0.25 D of power should be added to the contact lens.

Over Refraction

The power of the contact lens should preferably be calculated by doing over refraction (refracting over the trial contact lens). The final power, should be prescribed by adding algebraically the trial lens power and the acceptance over the contact lens. The over refraction should always be within 4 diopters so that the error due to the back vertex power is eliminated. The detail of power calculation is discussed in the fitting chapter.

9 The Initial Examination

A routine preliminary examination should be done for each patient before fitting contact lenses. The purpose of doing this is to:

1. Determine if the contact lenses are indicated or contraindicated
2. Record important information before CL wear to establish a base line and assess changes if any.

The initial examination consists of following steps:

1. Assess reasons for wanting contact lenses and the motivation
2. Take detailed history of patient's general condition, ocular condition, medication, and previous vision correction, occupational and environmental factors.
3. Evaluate patients refractive error and best corrected vision
4. Examine the eye

1. Assess **reasons for wanting contact lens** and motivation.
2. **Ocular examination:** Perform a complete ocular examination to rule out any abnormality. This is best done with a slit lamp. A torch with hand magnifier, or a 10 diopter lens case or a Burton lamp can also be used.

   These findings are necessary to indicate patient's suitability and prepare baseline findings.

   Assess the following structures: Rule out any abnormalities in the following:

   - Eyelid—like blephritis, meibomitis, trichaisis, chalazion, stye

- Bulbar and limbal conjunctiva—pinguecula, pterigium,
- Palpebral conjunctiva- papillae, concretions, cystic growth
- Cornea—any opacity, keratopathy, keratoconus, neovascularization
- Iris- iritis, iridectomy
- Tears—stability, viscosity, tearproduction , break up time
- Sclera—thinning.

3. Take a **detailed history of systemic conditions** and contact lenses: Some general conditions, which should be approached with caution while advising contact lenses, are
   - Diabetes—are prone to infections and have delayed healing
   - Pregnancy—prone to dryness and shift towards myopia, can continue lenses as long as they are comfortable
   - Allergies like asthma, hay fever –they are more prone to allergic reaction with solutions
   - Arthritis—may have handling problems if deformities happen, or associated with dryness
   - Sinusitis—more prone to red eyes and infections, more watering and discomfort.
4. **Previous contact lens wearer:** Careful history of his current contact lens and his satisfaction or failure should be evaluated to avoid repetition of such problems.
5. **Occupation and environment:** Knowing patients occupation and needs, help to suggest the best lens to the patient without dissatisfaction. Patients engaged in sports need very sharp vision and less moving lenses like the soft lenses. Certain daily needs and fine work requirement are deciding factor for the presbyopic patients. Patients in dusty environment may not adapt to RGP lenses and those in chemical industry may have burning and stinging problems with soft lenses.
6. **Refraction:** The next and the basic step before considering contact lenses is the refraction. The amount of the spherical

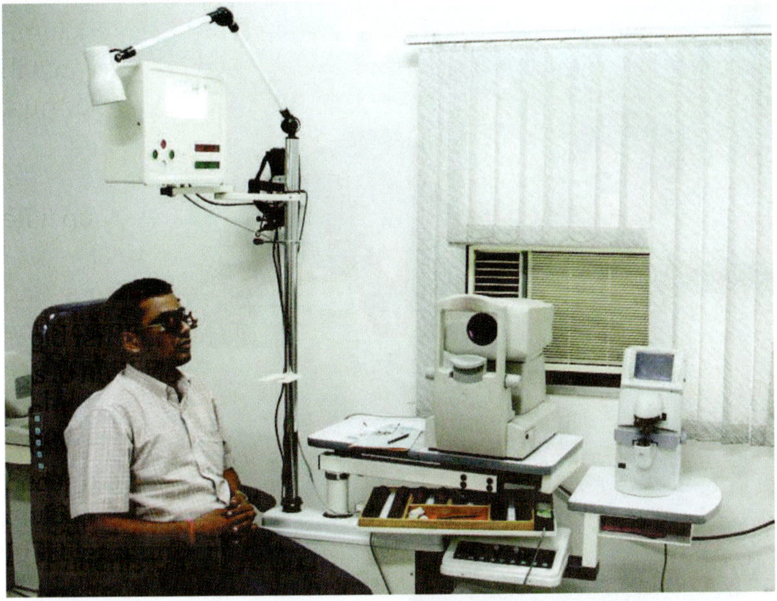

Fig. 9.1: Refraction

and cylindrical correction is also the deciding factor for selecting the type of the lens for the patient (Fig. 9.1).

Refraction and best-corrected visual acuity should be recorded. Vertex distance compensation should be made in case the powers are above +/–4.0 diopters. A Myope requires lesser power in contact lenses and a hyperope needs higher power in the lenses. Details of power calculations will be discussed later.

OCULAR MEASUREMENTS

Corneal Curvature—Keratometry (Fig. 9.2)

Corneal curvature is the basic and the most important measurement needed before starting contact lens fitting. The Keratometer measures only central 3 mm of the corneal curvature whereas the corneal topographer gives the complete mapping of the cornea. However the Keratometer measurement

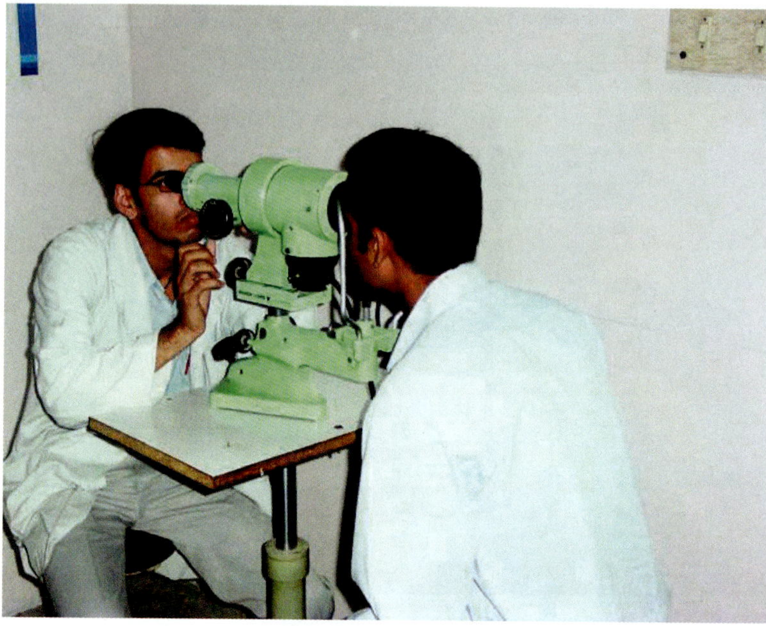

Fig. 9.2: Keratometry

is sufficient in most of the fittings. During the measurements one should also make note of the corneal irregularity if any.

The readings are taken in Diopters and then converted into millimeters. The readings also tell us about the degree of corneal astigmatism.

The base curve of the contact lens is determined by the corneal curvature measurements.

Corneal Diameter—HVID

Cornea is a curved surface so an easy way to measure its diameter is by measuring the HVID – horizontal visible iris diameter and the VVID – vertical visible iris diameter.

This measurement is taken by a simple millimeter scale , measuring the limbus to limbus size both across the horizontal and vertical lengths (Fig. 9.3).

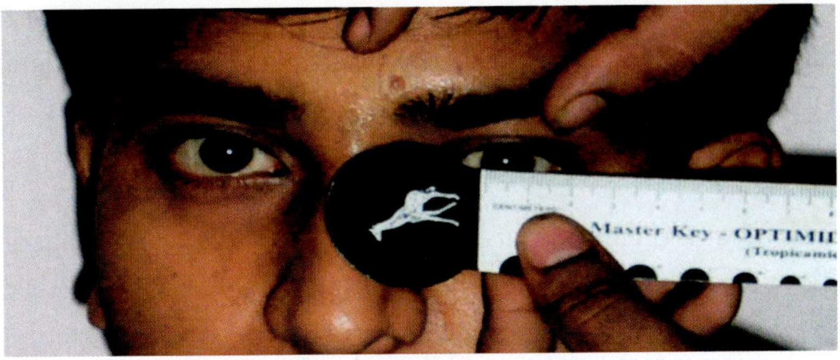

Fig. 9.3: Measurement of HVID

The corneal diameter aids in determination of the Total diameter of the contact lens.

Pupil Size

The diameter of the pupil is measured by a simple millimeter scale both in standard room illumination and low illumination. This aids in determining the optic zone size of the contact lens.

Palpebral Aperture and Lid Tension

The shape and size of Palpebral aperture varies in races specially the Asian versus Caucasian eyes. Measurements are done by millimeter scale. The main purpose is to record so that changes can be noted on follow-ups. There is no instrument to measure Lid tension.

It is a subjective method of measuring the tightness of the lid by asking the patient to look down and pinching the lids from the eyelashes. Tight lids indicate greater displacement of the lens and may lead to lid attachment fits. Lid tension can be classified as Tight, Loose and Medium.

Blink Rate

Normal blink rate (15 blinks per minute) is important for safe contact lens wear. Besides the recording of normal blink rate, the quality of the blinks, whether complete or partial should also be noted. Incomplete blinks will also lead to disrupted tear layer and corneal desiccation.

Tear Layer Assessment

Tear layer is an important aspect for estimating the suitability of the contact lens wear. The following tear layer measurements should be undertaken

- Schirmer test , phenol red thread test
- Break-up time
- Tear prism height
- Lipid layer evaluation.

Schirmer Test (Figs 9.4 and 9.5)

This test measures the volume of the tears. Special filter strips are bend over the notch and hooked over the nasal lower lid

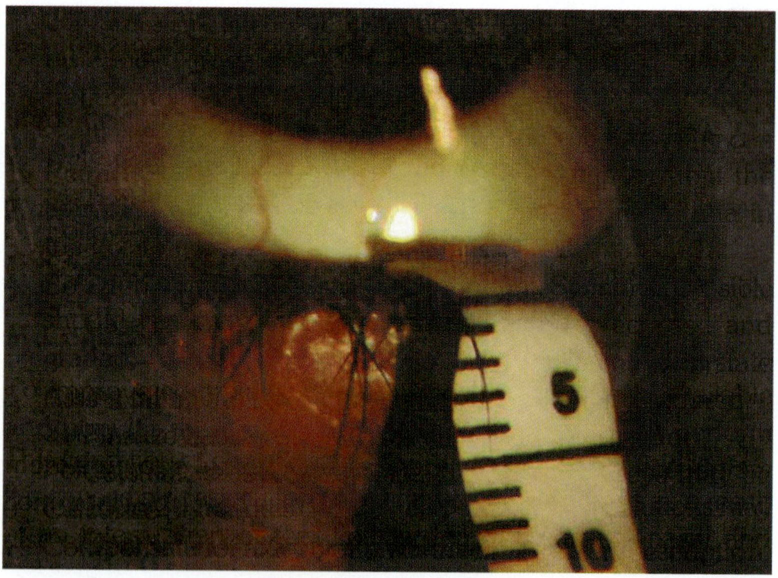

Fig. 9.4: Schirmers strip

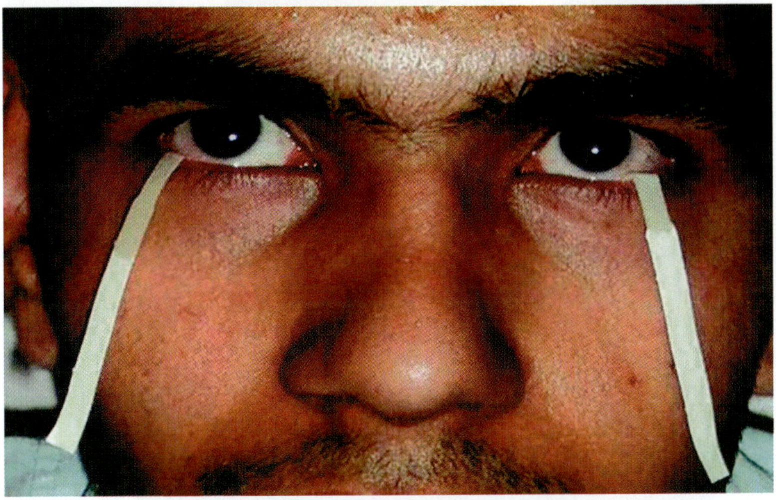

Fig. 9.5: Schirmers test

margin. Patient is asked to blink normal during the measurements. The wet area of the strip is measured after 5 minutes of insertion. Reading above 10 mm is taken as normal.

Phenol Red Thread Test

The test can be similarly done by using a 70 mm thread dipped in phenol red dye. The wet length is noted as color change from yellow to red.

Break-up Time

This test measures the stability of the tear film. Fluorescein dye is instilled in the eye and patient is asked to blink. The tear layer is then observed with the cobalt blue filter of the slit-lamp. The patient is now advised to hold blink and the time taken for the first dry spot seen on the cornea is measured in seconds. BUT - less than 10 seconds is suspicious of dry eye or unstable tear film (Figs 9.6A and B).

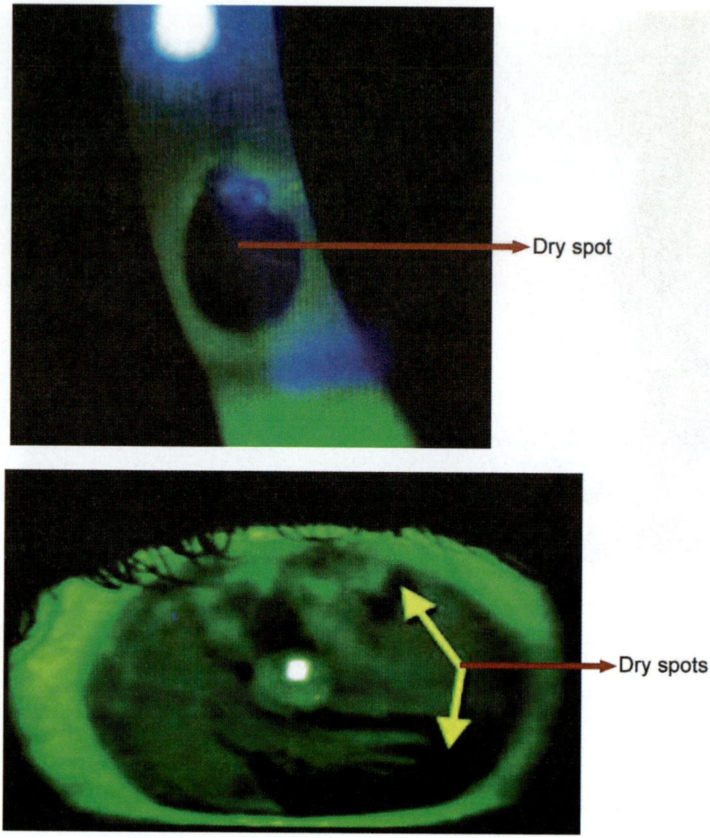

Figs 9.6A and B: Tear break-up time

The above is an invasive BUT time measurement. Avoiding fluorescein dye and just observing with the diffused illumination of the slit-lamp or by a Tearscope can also take non-invasive measurements.

Lipid Layer Evaluation

This is best done by the tearscope. Different colored fringes patterns are seen depending upon the thickness of the tear layer. Thicker the layer means better tear stability and less evaporation. Thicker layers also leads to lipid deposits problems.

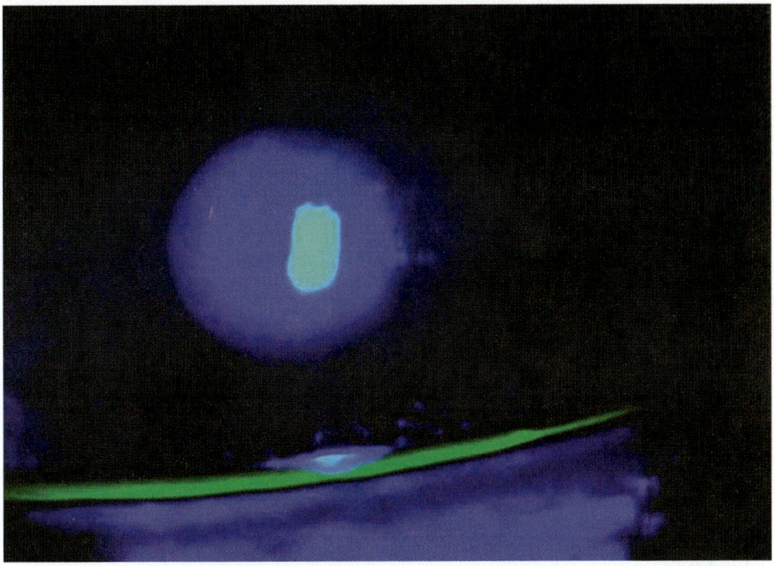

Fig. 9.7: Tear prism height

Tear Prism Height

This is the height of the tear reservoir seen at the lower lid margin. Normal tear prism heights range from 0.1 to 0.3 mm. Height less than 0.1 mm signifies dry eye (Fig. 9.7).

Patient's Specific Needs

The selection of the lens may vary according to:
- Patient's personal visual needs.
- Convenience and the duration for which the patient wants to wear lenses.
- Cost.

SUMMARY OF PRELIMINARY EXAMINATIONS

Recording History and Assessment of Indication/Contraindication

1. Indication for contact lens
2. Medical history any contraindication

3. Previous lens wear history
4. Motivation.

Ocular Examination

1. Visual acuity – uncorrected/ corrected
2. Refraction
3. Keratometry
4. Slit-lamp examination
5. HVID/VVID
6. Pupil size
7. Palpebral aperture
8. Lid tension
9. Tear break up time
10. Schirmer test
11. BUT
12. Suitability and type of lens.

10 Selection of the Lens—Options Available

There are several types of lenses and modalities; available in the market. It is practitioner's responsibility to decide the best lens for the patient. This section will discuss the various options available and how to choose the lens type for the patient.

Options of Lens Availability Based on Wear Modality

The lenses are classified according to the wearing modality

- Daily wear
- Extended wear
- Continuous wear
- Flexi wear

Daily wear: Lenses worn during waking hours, removed before the sleep period.

Extended wear: Lenses worn during sleep also usually continuously for six nights or *one week* and removed for cleaning and disinfection (not needed for weekly disposable lenses).

Continuous wear: Lenses worn continuously day and night for a continuous period from *one week to one month.*

Flexible wear: Lenses worn *for some days as extended wear* may be two or three nights and then shifted to daily wear. So it is an combination of extended and daily wear modality.

Selection of Wear Modality—Daily Wear vs Extended wear

Although all patients look forward to convenience of least maintenance and extended wear, still the safety of the eye should be the prime concern.

While selecting a lens for extended or continuous wear the lens should have sufficient oxygen transmissibility.

Both soft and RGP lenses are available as Daily or extended wear option. The following criteria should be kept in mind before deciding the modality for the patient.

Extended wear is a risky option if the patient's eye has following abnormalities

- Cornea—Edema, inflammation distortion, vascularization, opacities
- Tear film—signs of dryness, excess lipid
- Lid integrity—papillae or follicles
- Poor hygiene and compliance
- Higher powers (that increases the lens thickness at periphery or center)
- Previous history of complication with soft lens.

As far as possible, EW modality should be avoided because the incidence of the complications with contact lenses increases many folds when lenses are worn during sleep. Still there are conditions when the patients may need this modality like in

- Certain occupations
- Pediatric cases where it is not practical to insert and remove before and after every nap.
- Patient wants convenience or has handling problems.

The feasibility of EW or CW modality is getting more popular again, with the development of newer materials which are reducing the complications.

Classification on Basis of Lens Replacement Schedules

The lens needs to be replaced regularly mainly because it is not safe for the eye to use a lens that has warped, crazed, has scratches or is contaminated.

The lens replacement schedule for RGP and SCL are classified as:

RGP—Replacement

- Have longer life span and can be used up to 2-3 years till the lens starts creating problems like of blurred vision, irritation and foreign body sensation.
- The usual advise to the patient should be *one year* though
- The higher Dk RGP materials and EW RGP lenses however, need to be replaced more frequently.

SCL—Replacement Options are Classified as

- Conventional
- FRP—Frequent replacement program
- Disposable
- Daily disposable

Conventional lenses—are lenses, which replaced after they have lived their useful life. This is usually *one year.*

Frequent replacement—FRP or PRP planned replacement program lenses are those, which are replaced from a period of *1 month to 3 months.* These lenses follow the same care and maintenance regimen as conventional lenses. The so called monthly or quarterly disposable lenses actually fall under this category.

Disposable: These lenses are replaced every *week or two weeks.* The lenses need same care and maintenance except for the enzyme treatment.

Daily disposable: They are true disposable lenses which are discarded *daily* after every wear. The patient does not need any care and maintenance with these kind of lenses.

Selecting the Replacement Schedule for the Patient Depends Upon

- Conventional lenses for patients with normal ocular conditions and no signs of bad lid integrity, corneal changes or dryness.
- The earlier the lenses are replaced the safer they are for the eyes. Patients with any sign of abnormality should be suggested an early replacement program.
- Daily disposable are safest for the eye and can be advised to patients who need to wear the lenses on occasional basis. Patients sensitive to solutions are also suitable for this option
- Patients whose visual demands are high should dispose lenses frequently.
- Patients with lid changes specially GPC (giant papillary conjunctivitis) or CLPC (contact lens induced papillary conjunctivitis) due to previous lens wear should opt for FRP.
- Patients who intend to wear lenses for longer hours need to select FRP or disposable lenses.
- COST issues—frequently the lens is replaced higher is the cost. This issue should also be discussed with the patient after suggesting the best lens to them.
- Compliance—a non-complaint patient should be suggested a disposable or daily disposable lens.

Lens Options—Types Available

Besides selecting the wear modality and frequency of replacement, the type of the lens design, material most suitable to the patient is also selected .Let us recall some of the **options available on the basis of the design and material the lenses.**

- SCL – spherical, toric, bifocal, cosmetic lenses
- RGP – spherical, (toric and bifocal– not yet in Indian market), special designs for keratoconus and reverse geometry lenses
- Special types like the hybrid or X Chrome lenses

Comparison of soft and RGP lenses

Soft advantages	*RGP advantages*
Good initial comfort	Better vision
Suitable for occasional wear	Long-term lens—better physiology
Variable wearing time	Durable
No foreign body sensation	Less maintenance
Suitable for sports	Corrects regular and irregular astigmatism
Used to change eye colors	Less complications

Selecting the Patient for the Soft lens

In comparison to the Rigid lens the Soft lens is indicated for the following patients

- When *comfort* is the prime importance and the patient is a sensitive one. Although soft lenses are comfortable initially, yet studies have shown that the RGP lens also gives the similar comfort once adapted to.
- When the patient *wants immediate adaptation* and is nor willing to comply with the gradual adaptation of the rigid lens. This situation may also arise in cases where the patient has some occasion or purpose to wear lenses and does not have the time to wait and adapt to rigid lenses.
- When the patient wants to wear the lens *occasionally*. Rigid lenses should be worn regularly. If the patient discontinues wear for week or two with RGP lenses the initial sensations will revive and the patient will need to restart the adaptation schedule.
- Patients having *low refractive errors* will find it difficult to adjust to RGP lenses.

- *Sports person* who want greater lens stability should be advised soft lenses.
- Patients *in dusty and windy weather* conditions will have fewer problems, with soft lenses.
- If *eye color has to be changed* or opacities to be hidden, soft lens is the option.

Selecting the Rigid Gas Permeable Lens for the Patient

Even though the maximum fittings around the world, is the soft lens, yet there are indications where Rigid lenses are more suitable than soft lenses.

The RGP lens is a better indication than soft lens in the following situations

- *Astigmatism* which is not corrected by soft toric lenses also. Sometimes the prescriptions may be beyond the range of the manufacturers supply.
- Patients who give a history of recurrent difficulties or *Infections* with soft lenses
- All cases of *irregular astigmatism* Like keratoconus , corneal scars, traumatic corneas, etc. will benefit visually with RGP lenses only.
- Patients with *GPC are safer* with RGP lenses, though disposable lenses can also be used.
- Patients with *high refractive errors,* who have a possibility of hypoxia due to thick center or periphery, may be suggested high Dk RGP lenses
- Patients *with poor compliance and hygiene* are always at low risk of infections with RGP lenses.

Choosing the Most Suitable Lens (Table 10.1)

Following are some of the examples in **selecting the lens in specific eye conditions.**

Ultimately the practitioner should settle for the type of lens which best suits the patients needs.

Table 10.1: Selecting the lens in various eye conditions

Condition	*Lens type*	*Wear modality*	*Replacement modality*	*Remarks*
Low spectacle cylinder	SCL – spherical	DW/EW	Any	Cylinder upto 0.75 D or 4:1 ratio (sph:cyl), thick SCL
Medium spectacle cylinder	SCL –toric or RGP – spherical	DW	Conventional or FRP	SCL toric if spec cyl = K cyl
High Cylinder	SCL –toric RGP- sph	DW	Conventional FRP	SCL cyl up to 4 diopter only available
High Powers	RGP- high Dk SCL	DW	Any , prefer disposable for soft	SCL -High water content /Higher Dk/t /Non ionic
Dry *eye*	SCL	DW	Disposable/FRP	Low water thick Non ionic, medium Dk
High power/ cyl	RGP SCL	DW	FRP / Disposable	High water content SCL
Keratoconus	RGP	DW		Mid Dk special design
Irregular corneas/ irregular astigmatism	RGP- spherical	DW		High Dk
Therapeutic purposes	SCL	EW	Disposable/ continuous wear	High water content/ thin lenses/ High Dk

Selection of the Patient for the Contact Lens

Before proceeding for the contact lens fitting the practitioner must determine whether the patient is suitable for contact lens or not. Besides the visual indications the following criteria should also be considered after the initial examination is done.

1. *Motivation:* The patient will be a successful lens wearer only if the patient is self motivated to wear contact lenses. There may be some apprehension in beginners' mind, which can be taken care of by convincing them and overcoming their fears with lenses.
2. *Hygiene:* If the patient does not have a good personal hygiene he is not a suitable candidate for lenses. He may land up with infections which can be sight threatening at times.
3. *Compliances:* Some maintenance instructions may be outlined to the patient. The patient should be ready to comply to the instructions, the Do's and don'ts of the lens wear properly.
4. *Availability:* The refractive error of the eye should be within the range of the manufacturers supply.
5. *Refractive error:* Contact lenses are indicated for all types of refractive errors. The lenses are superior than the spectacles as they eliminate most of the aberrations, give wider field of vision and reduce aniseikonia. Lenses are the best option for anisometropia correction especially in unilateral aphakes. To eliminate irregular astigmatism lenses (rigid) is the only option. Lenses also reduce glare in albinism and aniridia. Nowadays lenses are available for presbyopes also.

It is the practitioner's responsibility to decide the best lens for the patient depending upon his needs.

11 Soft Contact Lens Fitting

It is a common feeling amongst most of eye care professionals that the soft contact lens fitting does not need proper skill. The fitting characteristic of soft lenses is a complex interaction of various ocular factors and definitely needs proper understanding of the fitting techniques. One has to also understand that it is the fitter's responsibility if the patient develops complications due to improper fitting.

To start with let us understand the **basic factors, which affect the fit of the lens on the eye.**

1. Soft lens has a very low **modulus of elasticity** and so it drapes the cornea, due to which it is generally seen that one universal base curve fits most of the corneas. Thin lenses are also more flexible, so they move less than the thicker lenses.
2. **Manufacturing method** creates a difference in fitting. Identical curvatures but different methods will cause different movement levels.
3. Fitting also depends upon the **water content**. Higher water content lenses are more flexible so will move less than the low water content lens (provided the thickness is the same).
4. **Keratometry readings** are never a true predictor of the corneal shape and the Sag values of the cornea. Thus patients with same K readings can have different lens parameters.
5. The movement of the lens fitting also depends upon the **eyelid forces and position.**
6. **Tear film** can also change the fitting characteristics. The lens tends to dehydrate on a dry eye and so will move less.

Ionicity also alters fitting, hypertonic tears cause lens to dehydrate and thus move less.

Considering all of the above factor, it is sure that one can go wrong in predicting a perfect lens for the patient on Empirical calculations. I suggest, one must evaluate the fitting on the trial lens method basis.

The Ideal Soft Contact Lens Fit

The overall goal of the soft lens fitting is to provide a lens, which gives adequate coverage, proper centering and adequate movement so that the tear exchange and the debris is not accumulated. The lens should not be tight on the eye so that it causes limbal compression, at the same time it should not be too loose to that it is uncomfortable and causes unstable visual acuity.

The Fitting Steps

i. Do initial examination of the eye on the slit lamp biomicrosope
ii. Determine the patient is suitable or not for soft lenses
iii. Do accurate refraction. The spectacle cylinder should not be more than 0.75 diopters or well within 4:1 ratio (spherical power : cylinder power)
iv. Measure the corneal curvature by Keratometer. Although Keratometer is not a true predictor of the soft lens base curve, as it has been studied that the fitting is dependent on the sag values and the shape factor of the cornea, yet K readings cannot be ignored. If, available corneal topography is more reliable.
v. Measure the HVID. The lens selected should be larger than the HVID.
vi. Carry out other routine examinations like tear film assessment.

vii. Select the lens type for the eye, Water content, material, thickness, modality, etc.

viii. The selection of the trial lens:

The soft lens has the following basic parameters. The parameters of the trial lens, is selected on the following criteria;

- Base curve
- Power
- Diameter
- Type of the lens.

Base Curve

Base curve is chosen on the basis of the keratometry. The modern designs may not actually predict the base curve, yet this is the only logical way of selecting the first trial lens for the eye. Typical base curves range from 8.1 to 9.1 mm (in 0.1 steps)

Steps for Calculations

1. Measure corneal curvature = convert in millimeters (refer to conversion chart)
2. Add 1 to the mean K reading
   For example, Km = 43.0 @180 /43.50 @90
   = 7.85 / 7.76
   = 7.80
   Add 1 to 7.80 = 8.80 mm
   This is the base curve of the trial lens needed to start with.

a. This is best true for thick lenses, thin lenses need lesser addition to K reading
b. Depend upon the manufacturer's guidelines in the fitting guide in trial lens selection.
c. Manufacturers nowadays usually do not supply curves in 0.1 increments. There may be 2 or 3 base curves available. Select the lens closest to the required BC.
d. Where only 2 base curves are available, select the steeper BC for steep cornea and Flatter BC for flat cornea.

Power/Back Vertex Power

The lens selected should have the power as close as possible to the spectacle power, or else maximum within +- 4 diopter of the spectacle power. Disposable lenses can be fitted by empirical calculation of the contact lens power based on the spectacle power.

Before fitting spherical soft lens one also needs to see that the spectacle cylinder is not more than 0.75 D. More than this may need a toric lens. (Detail of selection of toric lens will be discussed in toric chapter)

There are 3 basic steps to calculate the expected power of the soft contact lens.

i. Transpose into minus cylinder form
ii. Spherical equivalent calculation—Half the amount of cylinder and add to the spherical power (algebraically)
iii. Vertex distance calculation—If the spectacle prescription is more than 4.0 diopters. Power must be adjusted for vertex distance. This can be read from the tables. Spectacle lenses are usually 13 mm from the cornea and contact lenses are supposed to be at virtually zero distance from the cornea.

Some Examples

Spectacle power	*Remarks*	*Contact lens power (DS)*
–2.50 DS	Same as Sp Rx as less than 4.0 D	–2.50
–2.50 / -0.50 DC @180	Half the cylinder and add to spherical –2.50 + (–0.25)	–2.75
–8.0 DS	More than 4 , so refer to BVP chart	–7.25
–8.0 / –1.0 DS @ 90	Spherical equi = –8.50 Next compensate for vertex distance	–7.75
+ 2.0 / + 0.50 Dcyl @90	= +2.50/ –0.50@180= +2.25 (spherical equi)	+2.25

Selection of Power from Trial Sets

It is not possible to have all powers in all base curves. Unless, one stocks an inventory.

The **basic trial set** has the following powers in different base curves

1. –3.0 DS
2. –10.0 DS
3. +3.0 DS
4. +10.0 DS

The –3.0 lens works for all powers from 0 to –6.0 of spectacle prescription (within + – 4 diopters). The -10.0 lens is suitable for anywhere between –6.0 to –14.0. A + 3.0 lens will work from 0 to +6.0 and the +10.0 from +6.0 to +14.0.

After calculating the contact lens power from the spectacle prescription, select the trial lens with closest power or within 4 diopters of spectacle lens power. In case of disposable lenses, calculate empirically and select the lens from the inventory.

Diameter

The third basic parameter of soft lens is the diameter. *The diameter is selected on the basis of the HVID measurements. Add 2 mm to the HVID and the lens, diameter should be at least that much.*

Typical soft lens diameters range from 13.0 to 14.5 mm (in 0.50 steps). It is logical to have an observation of the cornea; normal corneal sizes can be fitted in this range. Smaller corneas may need smaller diameters and some extra large ones may need 15 mm. These unusual lenses are usually custom designed and are lathe cut designs. The basic rule is to cover the cornea adequately, so that there is no exposure of the limbus on blinks leading to discomfort and epithelial staining.

Lens Thickness

The lenses can be classified as

1. Thick—1 mm to 1.5 mm
2. Thin—0.5 mm to 1 mm
3. Ultra thin—< 0.6 mm

The selection will depend upon the following pros and cons:

Thick Lenses

1. Thick lenses are supposed to mask cylinders better than the thin ones.
2. Thick lenses are easier to handle and can be suitable for those who are likely to have handling problems.
3. Thick lenses reduce the oxygen transmissibility.

Thin Lenses

1. Have excellent transmissibility.
2. Drape the cornea so well that they do not mask astigmatism very well.
3. Have greater tendency to dehydrate and may cause corneal desiccation staining. This is more likely in ultra thin lenses.
4. They are not suitable for dry eyes.

Place the Trial Lens on the Eye (Figs 11.1 and 11.2)

Although the patient with soft lenses will adapt immediately yet one must wait for some time before evaluating the fit. This is because there is some amount of watering, and secondly the soft lens tends to loose some water when on the eye, which may lead to parameter changes.

It has been studied that it is best to assess the soft lens fitting 5 minutes after insertion. Waiting for 15 to 20 minutes is not essential for the fitting assessment, but sometimes more time may be given to the patients who want to psychologically adapt to them.

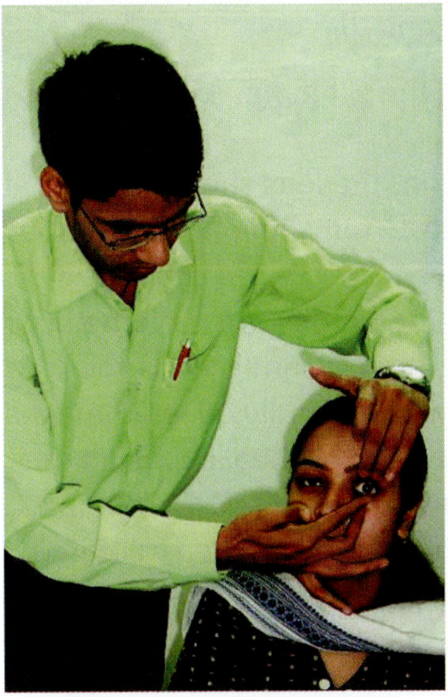

Fig. 11.1: Correct way of insertion of the trial lens

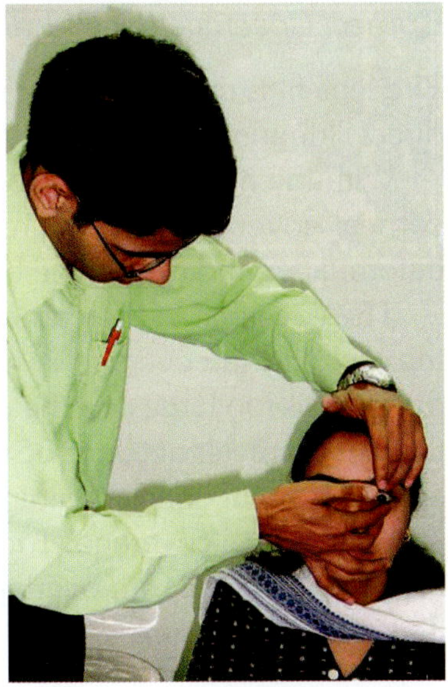

Fig. 11.2: Incorrect way of insertion of the trial lens

Evaluation of the Fit

Once trial lens has been fitted, its assessment has to be done. The following are the major criteria for fitting assessment.

Patients Comfort Response

There will be some awareness of the lens, but there should not be discomfort. Sometimes the initial discomfort is because of the differences of the lens solution pH and the tears. This resolves quickly (Fig. 11.3A and C).

Comfort is an initial clue to the fit assessment.

1. Fairly comfortable initially Probably good fit
2. Uncomfortable Predicts loose fit (because it moves too much)
3. Very comfortable May be steep or tight (because it is immobile)

Corneal Coverage (Figs 11.3E, F and J)

The lens fit is evaluated best with the slit lamp, using a diffuse direct illumination.

With the eye in primary position, the lens should show full corneal coverage about 1 mm to 2 mm beyond the limbus before, after and during the blink.

The coverage of the cornea is the predictor the diameter of the lens. If the coverage is more than 2 mm means the lens diameter is too large or if the cornea is not fully covered means the lens diameter needs to be increased. Corneal exposure may lead to corneal drying, staining and irritation.

1. Full corneal coverage (1 to 2 mm overlap) Ideal required
2. Greater than 2 mm overlap Lens too large
3. Corneal exposure Lens too small

Lens Centration

The lens should be reasonably centered, extending equal distance beyond limbus in all directions. This means that the optical center of the lens should fairly coincide with the center of the pupil. A decentered lens can cause blurred vision and discomfort. Some decentration with adequate coverage all around is acceptable. Decentered lens is not a true predictor of the tightness or looseness. It has to be judged by other methods also to decide what alteration has to be done.

1. Centered in all positions of gaze—Ideal and required (Fig. 11.3D)
2. Decentered with corneal exposure in any position of gaze—Lens may be tight or loose, diameter may be small. A thinner lens can be tried (Fig. 11.3G).

Lens Movement (Fig. 11.3H)

The movement of the lens is essential for proper tear exchange and removal of debris. Inadequate movement will lead to

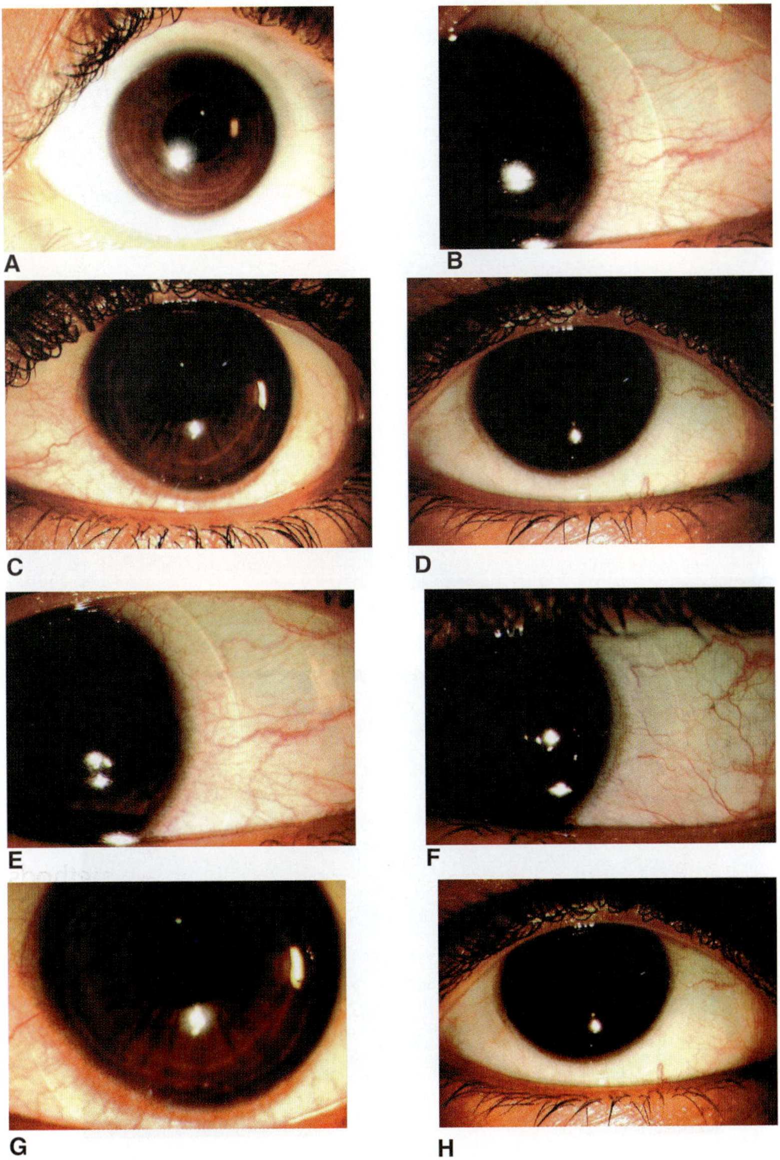

Figs 11.3A to H: (A) A comfortable soft lens, (B) Conjunctival indentation with tight lens, (C) An uncomfortable lens, (D) Centered lens with complete coverage in all positions of gaze, (E) Full corneal coverage, (F) Excess coverage, (G) Decentered lens, (H) Assess movement in primary gaze and blink

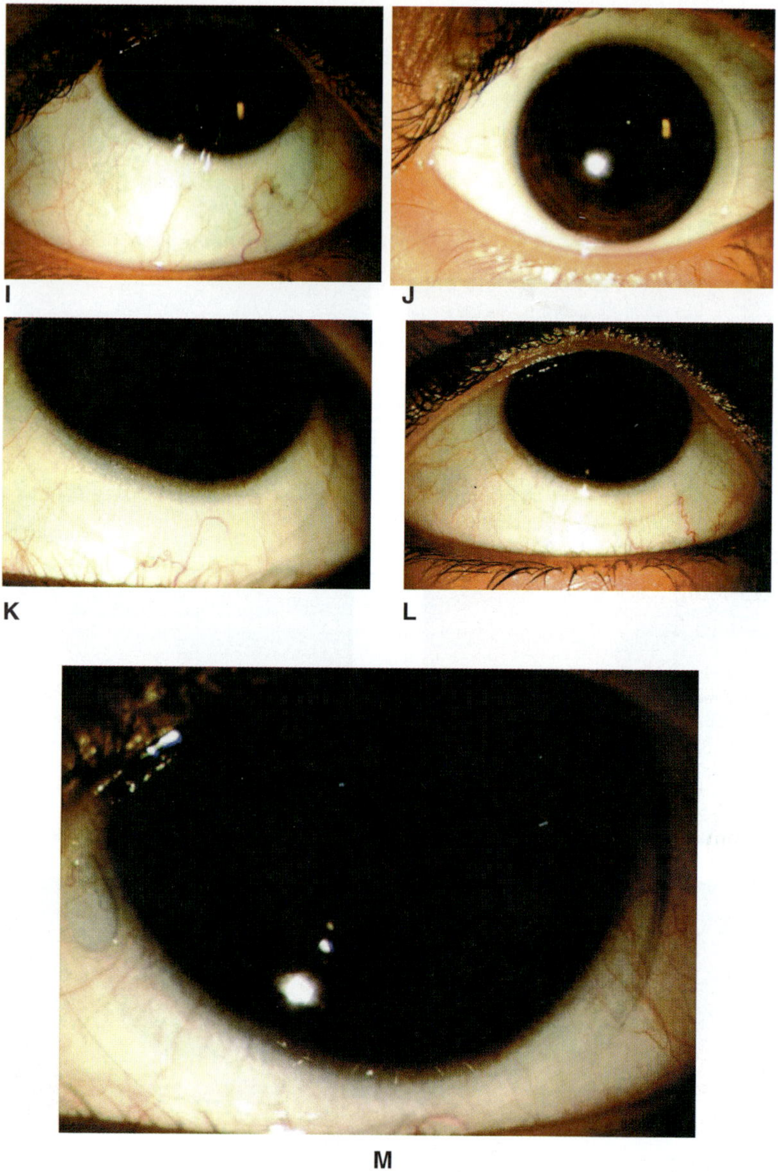

Figs 11.3I to M: (I) Excess lag in flat lens, (J) Improper coverage and exposure, (K) Lag on upgaze, (L) Less lag in steep lens, (M) A steep lens with bubble and conjunctival indentation

inflammation, edema and red eye (CLARE). It is the most important evaluation technique.

The movement of the lens is a judgment of an individual. The patient is asked to look straight in the primary gaze and asked to blink normally. Estimate the movement of the lens while observing with diffuse light and high magnification the amount of the movement with each blink. The best way is to learn from experience initially by trying different base curve lenses on an individual and estimating the steepness and flatness on the basis of the movement.

The movement of the lens depends upon the type of the lens, its design and thickness. One must follow manufacturers guidelines. Thick lathe cut lenses may need a movement of 1 to 2 mm, but modern thin design lenses are required to move by 0.2 mm to 0.1 mm This small movement of the lens is at times difficult to assess. The *push up test* is always performed with this to finally decide if the lens is steep or flat.

0.2 to 0.4 mm movement	Ideal movement	For thin lenses
> 0.2 mm movement	Tight lens	For thin lenses
< 0.4 mm movement	Loose lens	For thin lenses
1 mm to 2 mm movement	Ideal	For thick lenses

Push-up Test

Push-up test is a valuable aid in determining the lens fitting relationship.

The patient looks straight and the examiner pushes the lens up vertically, through pressure on the lower lid (Fig. 11.4).

The examiner will then estimate the relative ease with which the lens moves up and the smoothness by which it recenters.

A 100% tight lens will resist any movement on push and will be difficult to displace. A loose fitting lens will slide off easily but will be sluggish to return or may not recenter even.

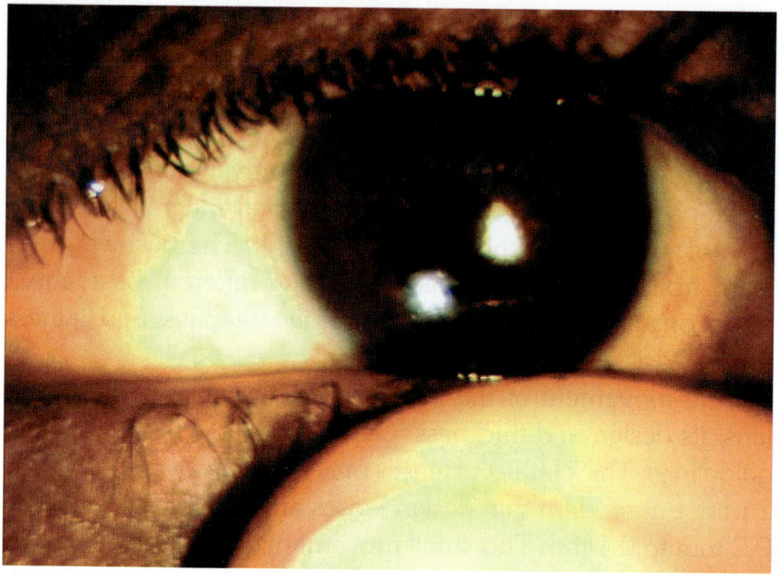

Fig. 11.4: Push-up test

An ideal fitting lens will displace easily and return smoothly. The tightness experienced on push-up test should be more than 50%. This again is a subjective judgment.

Easy displacement	Smooth recovery and recentration	Optimum fit
Resistance to displacement	May not recenter	Tight fit
Easy displacement	Erratic recovery	Loose fit

Lens LAG on Upgaze (Figs 11.3I, K and L)

The patient is asked to look up, the lens will move down slightly. This is called Lag. The amount of lag depends upon the fitting relationship.

An optimum fit shows a lag of 1 to 1.5 mm. Less than this indicates steep fit more than this indicates a flat fit.

Edge Alignment (Figs 11.3B and M)

The edge of the lens should be observed with reference to the conjunctiva. If the edge is sliding smoothly and aligning with the conjunctiva it is a desired result. If the lens edge indents on the cornea the lens is tight. If it stands off the lens is loose.

Other Responses for Estimation of Fitting Relationship

These are some more indicators in fitting assessment. Slight steepness and looseness cannot be predicted by these tests. Gross fitting errors can be estimated by them.

Vision Before and After Blink

If the lens fit is ideal the vision will remain clear before and after blink. Variation of vision with blink indicates steep or flat fit. If the vision clears with blink it is a steep fit, if it blurs after blink it is a flat fit.

Keratometry and retinoscopy with the lens on the eye can also be performed. The patient is asked to blink and the clarity of the mires soon after blink is observed. If it gets clear with blink it is a steep lens, if it gets blurred or distorted soon after blink it is a loose lens.

Alter the lens if ideal fit is not achieved

If the first trial lens does not show adequate fit, find and refit another appropriate lens.

There are 3 basic parameters on which the lens fitting depends.

The fitting relationship can be changed on this basis:

1. Base curve
2. Diameter
3. Thickness

Increasing the **base curve** flattens the lens fit and decreasing it steepens it. If 8.3 BC is behaving steep, depending upon the steepness, decide the next flatter BC like 8.4 or 8.5

Increasing the **diameter** increases the Sag so it tightens it. The diameter of the lens should be also be increased or decreased depending on the corneal coverage. Suppose a 14.5 mm diameter lens behaves tight reducing the diameter to 14.0 or 13.5 mm will flatten the fit.

Increasing the **thickness** of the lens fit increases the movement, hence loosens the fit.

Altering the base curve and the diameter—without changing the fitting relationship

The rule of thumb is

0.3 mm change in the base curve = 0.5 mm of change in diameter

Let us consider an example: an 8.3 mm BC , 13.5 mm lens will give the same fitting relationship as an 8.6 mm BC and 14.0 mm lens.

Bausch and Lomb—Series Lenses Fitting Principle

The parameter of thickness variation is utilized in the Series lenses of the Bausch and Lomb lenses. The series lenses are available as B, U, and O. Further classified as B3, B4 , U3, U4, O3, O4. Here 3 stands for 13.5 mm diameter and 4 stand for 14.5 mm diameter. B, U, and O signify the thickness. B-being a thicker lens series, U–further thin and O further thinner. If suppose, one fits a B3 lens and it is found to behave flat or loose on the eye, the next choice of lens to steepen it will be either a thinner lens or an larger lens. So the choice can be shifted to B4 or U3 lens. The diameter again can be judged from the corneal coverage. Each lens series also has a Sag value specified. The fits can be given on the basis of the sag values, a higher Sag means steeper fit and lesser Sag, means flatter fit.

Over Refraction

It is advisable to refract over the diagnostic lens to confirm the power of the lens and to rule out any residual astigmatism. The lens will also confirm the final visual acuity that can be achieved by the soft lens.

Do retinoscopy over the trial lens. Take patients acceptance by which it achieves the best visual acuity.

Calculate the final lens power by algebraically adding the power of the diagnostic lens and the additional power needed.

Note

a. The additional power needed should be always less than 4 diopters. (Else the back vertex calculations of the added lens will further have to be calculated)

b. The final lens power in the spherical lens fitting is a spherical power. So the additional lens power should always be spherical power. If there is significant cylindrical acceptance over the diagnostic lens and the vision is not acceptable by spherical equivalent then fit a toric lens.

Example:

Power of trial contact lens on the eye = –3.0 Dsph
Over refraction = +0.50 Dsph
Final lens power to be ordered = +2.50 Dsph

Final Order of the Soft Contact Lens

- Base curve
- Power
- Diameter
- Water content
- Tint
- Material
- Manufacturer

SUMMARY

1. Measure
   — Keratometry
   — HVID
2. Determine contact lens parameters
   — Base curve
   — Diameter
   — Power
3. Select the lens type
4. Assess fitting after lens settles on the eye
   — Coverage
   — Centration
   — Movement
   — Comfort
   — Push up test
   — Lag
5. Assess vision
   — Over refraction

Provide a lens that gives comfort and vision but is not tight on the eye.

12 RGP—Rigid Lens Fitting

Rigid lens fitting is more complex than the soft lens fitting. One has to have clear understanding of the lens design before learning the fitting. It takes real skill to fit the rigid lens to contour the individual's cornea. *The judgment of the fitting evaluation becomes better and better with experience and practice.*

The following chapter will try to explain the fitting criteria of RGP lenses. Once done it will be realized that the fitting of a rigid lens is as simple as a soft lens is.

The Rigid lens Parameters

Before starting, let us again have a look at the rigid lens design.

The lens parameters that need to be finalized for an individual eye are

- Base curve
- Power
- Diameter
- Optic zone
- Optic zone diameter
- Peripheral curve radius/width
- Center thickness
- Edge design
- Tint
- Material

The Ideal RGP Lens Fit

The rigid lens fitting is evaluated in two ways

1. **Static**—With the lens in stationary position, the fluorescein pattern with central alignment, mid peripheral minimal

clearance and adequate pooling in the peripheral curves is evaluated.

2. **Dynamic**—Evaluates the movement of the lens with the blink and further judge the tear exchange under it is called the dynamic fitting evaluation. The centration and the coverage are also evaluated.

Centration

A well-centered lens will remain on the cornea in all positions of gaze. The optic zone of the lens should cover the visual axis or the pupil of the eye throughout. If they don't then the wearer will have glare and ghost images. The decentered lens, which touches the conjunctiva, may also lead to staining and discomfort.

If the lens is well aligned with the cornea it will center well, otherwise the lens may be low riding or high riding (Figs 12.1A to C).

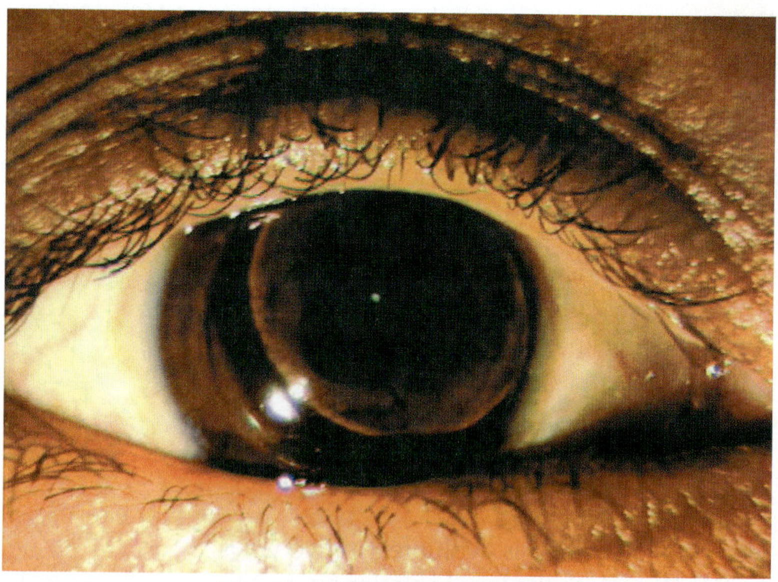

Fig. 12.1A: Well-centered lens

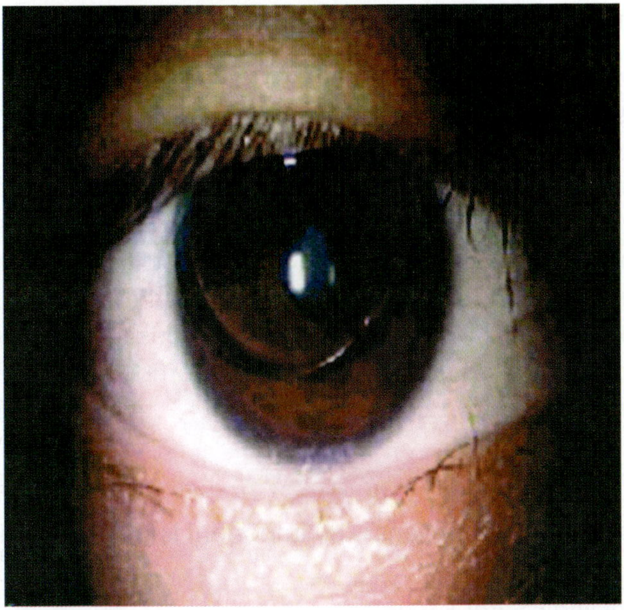

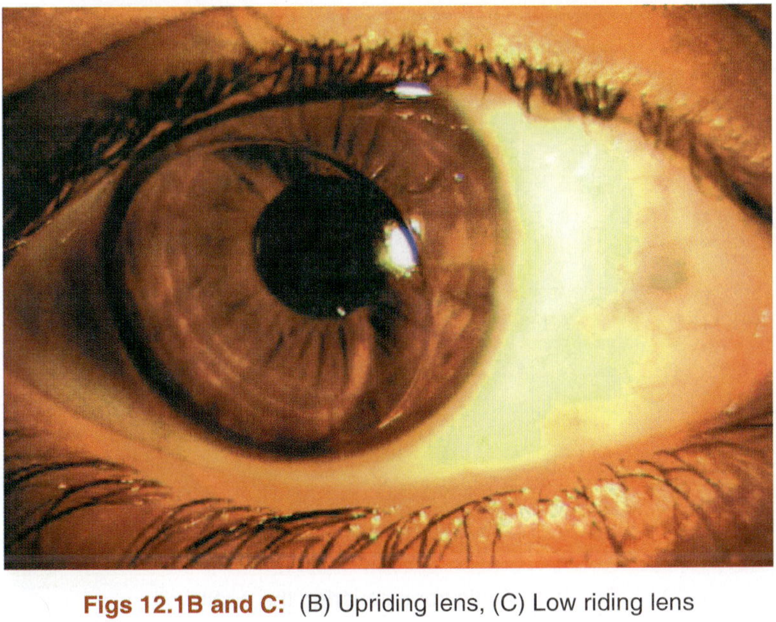

Figs 12.1B and C: (B) Upriding lens, (C) Low riding lens

Coverage

The rigid lens is smaller than the cornea unlike soft lens which are bigger and drape the cornea and the limbus.

The rigid lens is about 1.4 mm smaller than the HVID so that they can facilitate smooth tear exchange under the lens with each blink. The lens diameter should be such that it should be smaller than the cornea and should not reach the limbus. The diameter should also be not so small that the pupil does not cover the optic zone properly else will cause vision problems (The optic zone diameter is directly proportional to the overall diameter size) (Fig. 12.2).

Movement

The movement of the lens is an important issue in the rigid lens fitting because:

a. It facilitates tear exchange

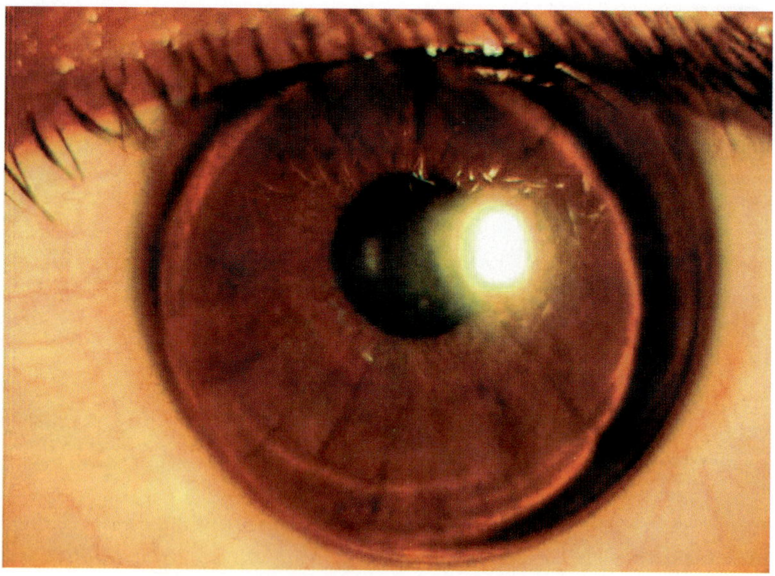

Fig. 12.2: Optic zone covering the pupil well

b. It removes the debris under the lens
c. There is significant exchange of oxygen underneath the RGP during blink.

An ideal rigid lens will move 1 to 1.5 mm vertically with each blink. This movement should also be smooth indicating an alignment fit.

- A steep lens will move less; will lead to stagnation of debris under the lens and hence staining and red eye.
- An excessively moving lens may be flat, will be uncomfortable to wear and will show variable vision (Fig. 12.3).

Alignment—Fluorescein Pattern

The ideal RGP lens should show alignment of the back surface of the lens with the cornea over most of the surface. The alignment of the lens back surface allows maximum tear exchange with minimum pressure over the cornea.

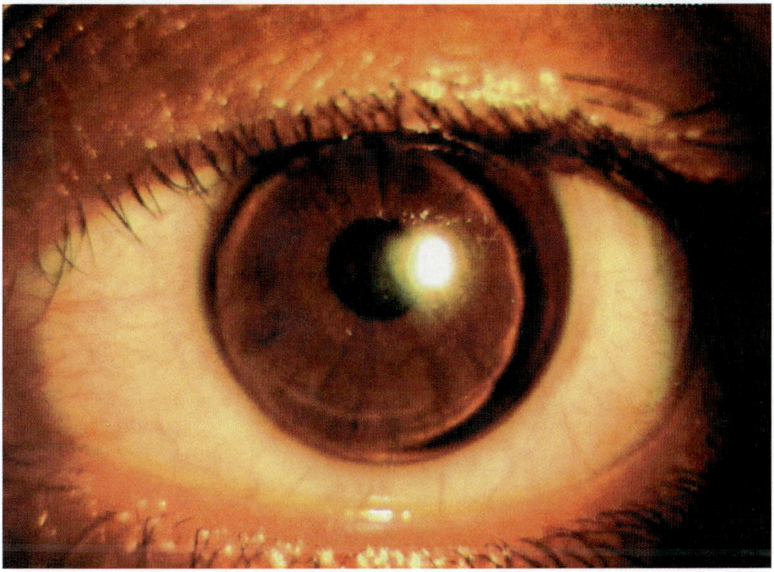

Fig. 12.3: RGP lens observe movement with blink

This alignment is best evaluated by the fluorescein pattern. The following are the *3 areas of observation* to define an ideal alignment fit—steep or flat on the eye.

- Central
- Mid-peripheral
- Edge width with clearance

Ideal Fluorescein Pattern (Figs 12.4A and B)

- Centration—central
- Movement—1 to 1.5 mm smooth
- Central—alignment
- The mid-peripheral bearing—minimal
- Edge band—0.26 to 0.35 mm

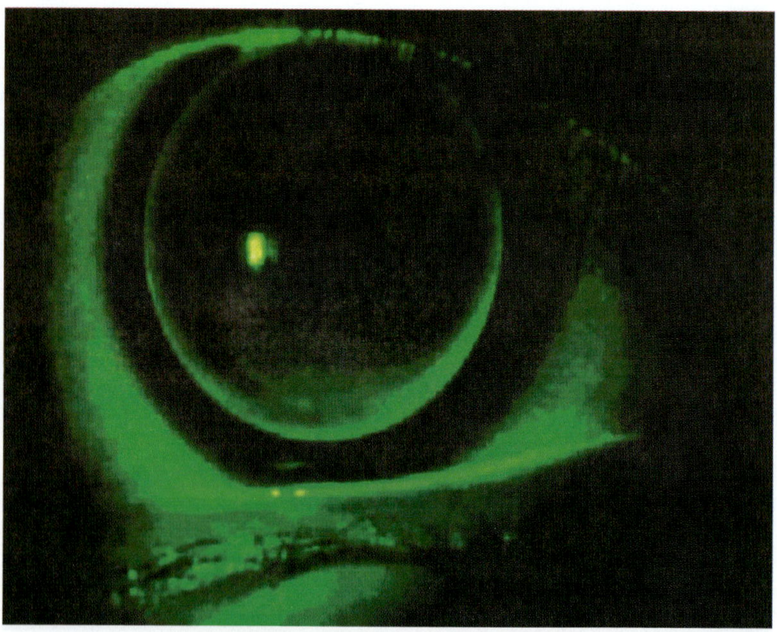

Fig. 12.4A: Ideal fluorescein with filter

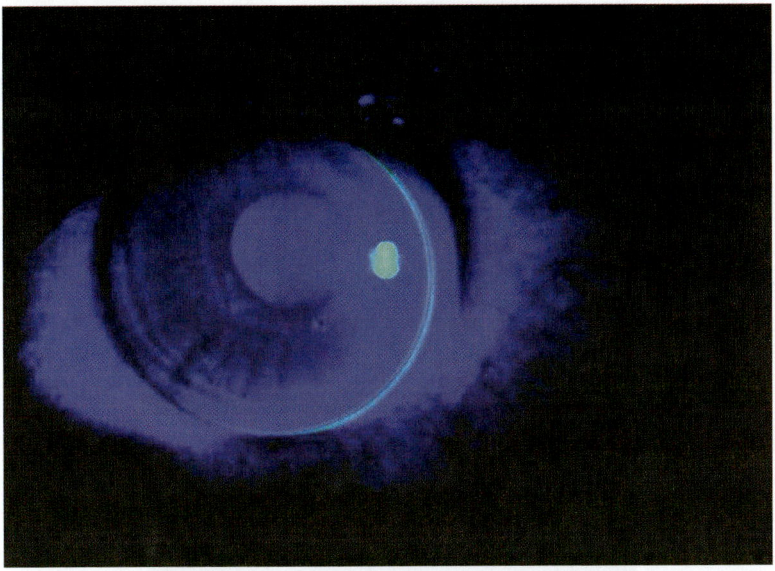

Fig. 12.4B: Ideal fluorescein pattern

Steep (Figs 12.5A and B)

- Centration—central
- Movement—restricted
- Central—pooling
- Mid-peripheral bearing—heavy
- Edge band—narrow < 0.25 mm

Flat (Figs 12.6A and B)

- Centration—poor, unstable
- Movement—excessive, rotation
- Central—touch
- Mid-peripheral—pooling
- Edge band—wide > 0.4 mm

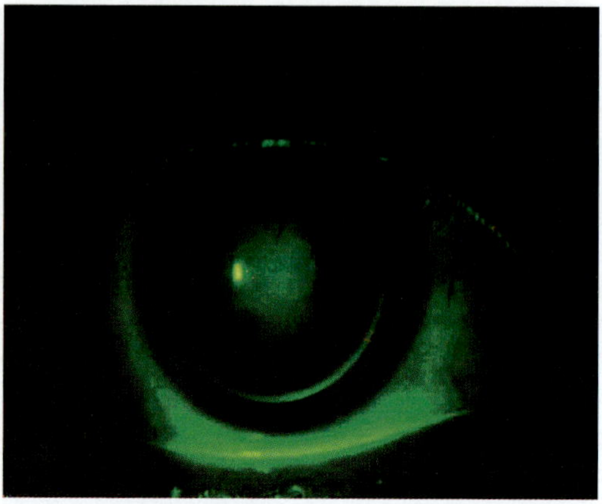

Fig. 12.5A: Steep fluorescein pattern

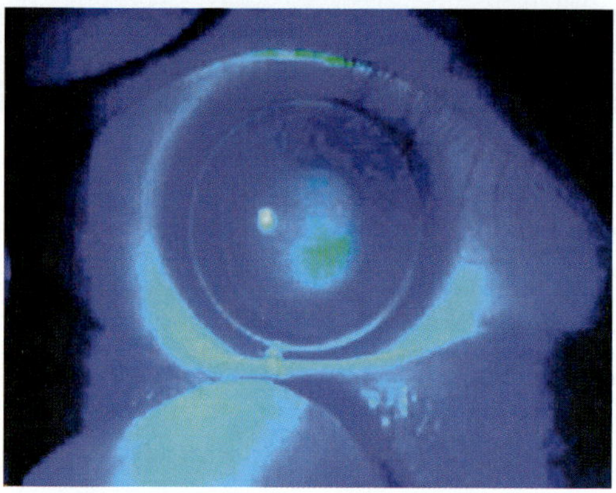

Fig. 12.5B: Steep fluorescein pattern

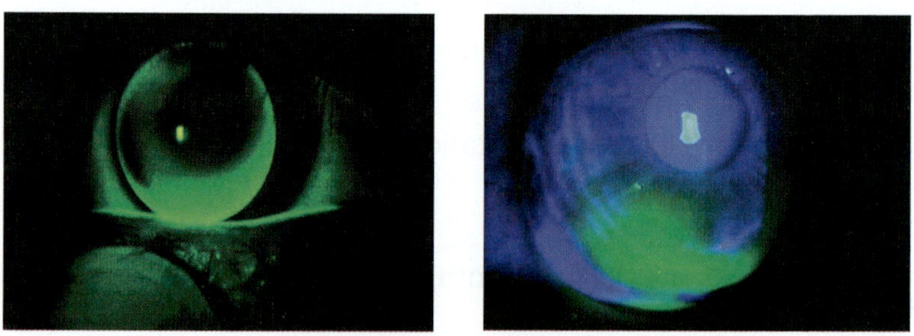

Figs 12.6A and B: Flat fit

PROCEDURE FOR RGP FITTING

Measure

Keratometry

Measure the flattest and the steepest corneal curvature using the Keratometer. It is indispensable. The Base curve of the trial lens is selected on this basis. The back curve of the lens has to align with the corneal curvature, so measure the K readings with maximum accuracy. K readings should be taken as mean of 3 readings.

The central 3 mm readings are usually sufficient to decide the fitting. There may be corneal shapes at times that may create variations in fitting. In that case peripheral readings or topography is important.

Refraction

Best corrected spectacle prescription in minus cylinder form need to be confirmed before fitting lenses.

Tear Quality

Assess the tear quality. Integrity of the tear film is important for the tolerance and fitting status of the lens.

Type of Astigmatism Affects Lens Choice

Spherical RGP can neutralize the corneal astigmatism. Better success is achieved vision wise for with the rule astigmatism. The lenticular astigmatism can be best corrected by Front surface toric RGP or soft toric lens.

HVID

Measure the horizontal visible iris diameter with the help of a ruler. This is used to choose the initial total diameter of the lens. It is 1.2 to 1.4 mm smaller than the HVID.

Pupil size

Measure the pupil size in low and average illumination. The size of the optic zone needs to be larger than this.

TRIAL LENS SELECTION

First of all the trial lens set from which the first diagnostic lens has to be chosen should be of the same manufacturer whom one is going to order. Each manufacturer has its own design and curve dimensions which will make difference if a different manufacturer makes it. Many a times the optic zone diameter, peripheral curves design is ordered same as in the trial lens if the trial fit is satisfactory. These are precalculated according to the base curve, diameter, power and the material selected. There may be times when the secondary curves and the zone need to be specified, in cases where the corneal shape deviates from the normal population.

The Trial Sets

The manufacturer's trial sets have base curves in 0.25 D (0.05 mm) difference. The power of the trial lens is usually –3.0 D sph. The diameter is pre calculated, according to the design by the manufacturer, usually ranging from 9.0 to 9.6 mm. The larger diameters are chosen for the flatter base curves and the smaller diameters for the steeper base curves.

One needs to have 3 more trial sets with powers –10.0 D, +3.0, +10.0 D. The variation in base curves in these 3 sets can be in 0.50 diopter (0.1 mm).

Selection of the Lens

From the measurements of the eye taken, select the trial lens from the appropriate trial set. The selection criterion is as follows:

Base Curve

- Depends on the Keratometry readings and the corneal astigmatism

- K stands for flatter corneal curvature reading
- The following table is the general guide. One must refer to manufacturers guide also before selection

K and astigmatism (if astigmatism is ..	*Base curve selection*	*Example*	*Base curve selected (chose closest from trial set available)*
0 – 0.75 D	Fit on K	41.0(8.23): 41.50(8.13)	8.23 mm
0.50 – 1.0 D	Fit on 0.05 mm steeper than K	41.0 (8.23): 42.0 (8.04)	0.05 mm steeper than 8.23 mm = 8.18 mm (41.25)
1.0 – 2.50 D	Fit 0.10 mm steeper than K	41.0(8.23): 43.0 (7.85)	0.1 mm steeper than 8.23 = 8.13 mm (41.50)
> 2.50 D	Fit on mean Keratometry readings	41.0 (8.23): 44.0 (7.67)	Mean K =7.94 mm (42.50 D)
Higher corneal astigmatism	May need toric lenses		

Overall Diameter Selection

The overall diameter is selected on the following criteria

- HVID—usually 1.2 to 1.4 mm smaller than the HVID
- Base curve—flatter base curves usually need larger diameters, steeper go well with smaller diameters.
- Astigmatism—smaller lenses improve comfort for high astigmatisms (> 2.50 Ds)
- Palpebral aperture and the lid position
  - Smaller palpebral aperture—smaller diameter 9.0 to 9.2 mm
  - Larger Palpebral aperture—larger diameters 9.6 to 10 mm
  - Normal range—9.2 to 9.6 mm.

Power of the Trial Lens

Calculate the expected power of the contact lens from the spectacle prescription. *Select the trial lens within 4 diopters of this calculated power.*

Although it is best to be closest to the spectacle power, yet it is not practical to stock all powers and base curves in trial lenses. Agreed there may be some variation in central thickness of the final lens made due to difference in the power ordered, but that usually is overcome if the power is within 4 diopters of the trial lens. Use a plus power lens for hyperopes and high minus power lens for high myopes.

Perform over refraction in case of RGP lenses to finalize the power of the lens. One may go wrong if the over refraction is above + – 4.0 diopters.

How to Estimate Contact Lens Power in RGP Bases on Spectacle Prescription

Spectacle prescription	*Rule*	*Spectacle Rx example*	*Calculations steps*	*CL power (if fitted on K flatter reading)*
Spherical and < 4 .0 D	Same as Sp Rx	–2.50 Ds		–2.50
Sph/cyl and sph < 4.0 D	Transpose in minus cylinder form and drop the cyl	1. –2.50 D/ –1.0cyl @180 2.–2.50 Ds / +1.0 Dc@ 180	1. drop the cyl 2. transpose –1.50 DS/ –1.0 Dc @90 (then drop cyl)	–2.50 Ds 1.50 Ds
Spherical and more than 4.0 diopters	Refer to back vertex chart	–8.0 DS	–8.0 = -7.25 by vertex chart	–7.25 Ds
More than 4.0 Ds and plus cylinder	Transpose and then refer to BV chart	+10.0 / + 2.0 Dc @180	+12.0 / –2.0 Dc @ 90+12.0 (drop cyl)+14.0 (back vertex power)	+14.0 Ds

All these above calculations are the expected powers if we finalize the lens fitting on K (K = flatter curvature).

Remember to add power for the change in curvature if made in the final lens (Fig. 12.7).

For steepness = add minus power

For flatness = add plus power

The over refraction should also be done over the trial lens which is discussed later.

Other Parameters: Optic Zone, Peripheral Curves

One has little control over them during trial lens selection.

Optic Zone is

- 2 mm larger than pupil (dim light).

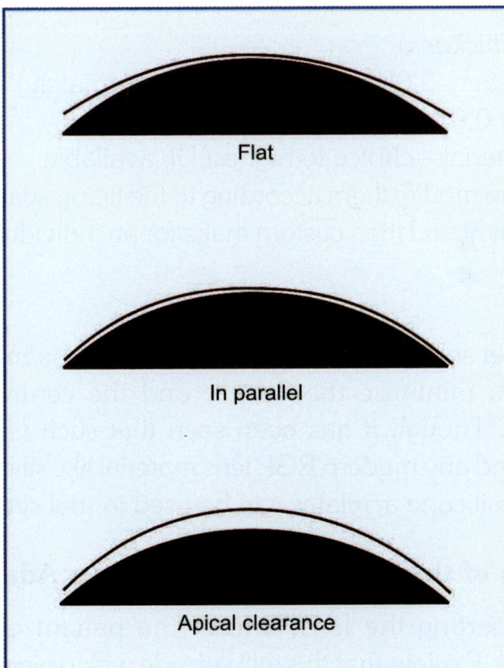

Fig. 12.7: Tear lens between cornea and lens (add power for change in curvatures)

Overall diameter	*Optic zone diameter*
9.0 to 9.2 mm	7.8 mm
9.3 to 9.5 mm	8.0 mm
9.6 to 9.8 mm	8.2 mm

Peripheral Curves are usually

- 1st—1.0 mm flatter than BC
- 2nd—2.0 mm flatter than BC
- 3rd—3.0 mm flatter than BC

Peripheral Curve width
- Usually 0.3/0.4 mm
- Depends on number of PC and OD

Central Thickness
- For power –3.0D = 0.15 mm (approximately)
- Modify 0.01 mm per diopter
- Dk material—choice to highest Dk available

One can modify them according to the fitting evaluation done on the patient and then custom make for an individual if needed.

Material

The trial set should be theoretically of the same material to be ordered to minimize the flexure and the central thickness variations. Though it has been seen that such variations are minimal and any modern RGP lens material like silicon acrylates and fluorosilicone acrylates can be used in trial sets.

Insertion of the Lens on the Eye and its Adaptation

Before inserting the lens, inform the patient of the initial discomfort. Explain that this will subside with usage and it takes a few days to get adapted to them.

The major discomfort with the rigid lens wear is due to the

interaction of the upper lid with the lens edge. Instruct the patient to look down with chin up for initial 5 minutes of the lens wear. Once his confidence builds up, let him look up.

Wait till the patient adapts and the watering stops, before evaluating the fit. This may take 20 to 30 minutes.

ASSESSMENT OF FIT

With a Torch or Diffuse Illumination and White Light of Slit-lamp

Evaluate the centration and the movement of the lens with the blink in primary gaze and lateral gaze with the white light.

Remember a flat lens will move excessive and the steep lens will show restricted movement. A steep lens may show good centering whereas a flat lens may be unstable and decentered. An air bubble trapped under the lens indicates a very steep fitting. Change the lens accordingly.

Once satisfied, proceed for the fluorescein evaluation.

Fluorescein Evaluation

Using a Burton lamp or the slit-lamp and cobalt blue light the Fluorescein pattern is observed. Minimal amount of the dye is inserted in the conjunctival sac with the help of Fluorescein strips and patient is then asked to blink. Care should be taken that excess dye is not inserted in the eye and also the eye is not watering (Fig. 12.8).

A Wratten filter # 12 can be used along with the blue light to enhance the contrast of and hence easy evaluation.

Observe these three areas under the lens:

1. Central
2. Mid peripheral
3. Edge

The amount of steepness and flatness has to be judged on the following basis. It needs experience and skill to grade the

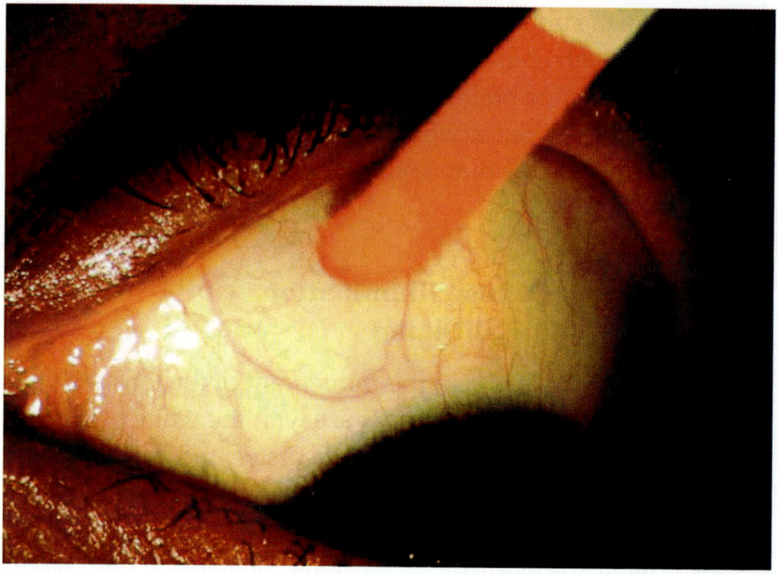

Fig. 12.8: Inserting dye with fluorescein

amount of steepness or flatness one needs to go into. This is not difficult at all and needs a little bit of experience and practice (Figs 12.9A to E).

	Ideal	*Steep*	*Flat*
Central fit	Alignment (uniform thin film of Fluorescein)	Central pooling (bubbles if excessive steep	Central touch
Mid-peripheral fit	Minimal or no contact	Touch or bearing	Pooling
Peripheral	Optimal band width of 0.2 to 0.3 mm Moderate clearance at the edge	Narrow band width < 0.2 mm Dim or no fluoro-scein at the edge	Wide band width >0.36 mm Bright fluorescein at the edge, bubbles may be observed if excessive flat

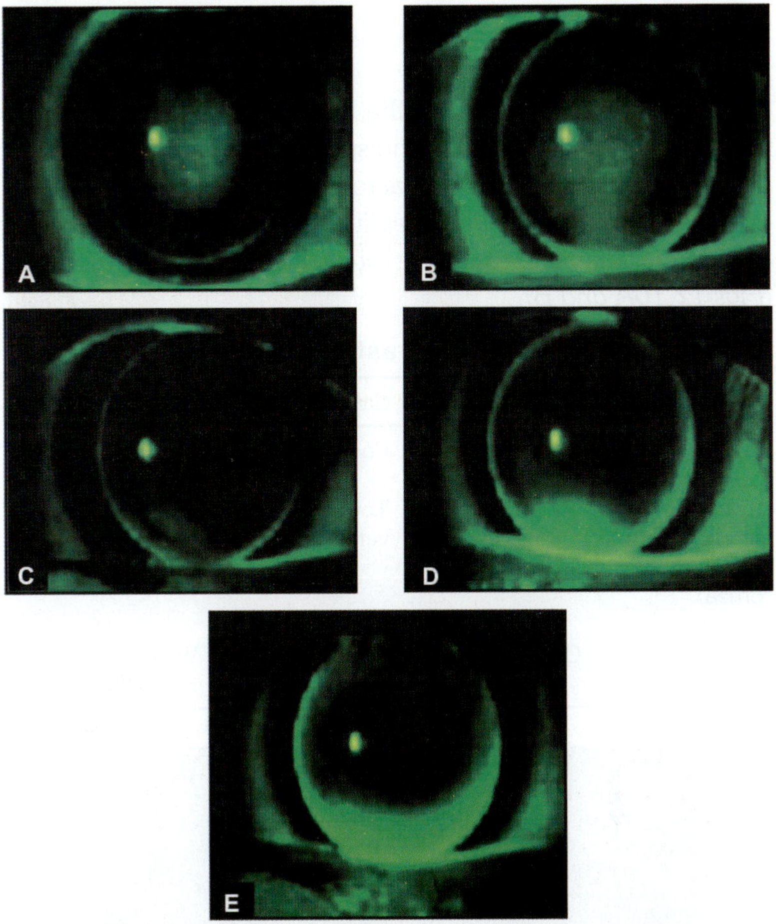

Figs 12.9A to E: Fluorescein patterns: (A) Very steep fit, (B) Steep fit, (C) Ideal fit, (D) Flat fit, (E) Very flat fit. **OBSERVE:** Fluorescein patterns at the edge: (A) Narrow edge of very steep fit, (B) Steep fit edge, (C) Ideal edge, (D) Flat fit edge, (E) Very flat fit edge

Spherical RGP on Astigmatic Cornea —Fitting Guide

Due to toricity of the cornea the mid-periphery and the edge pattern will be different than the spherical corneas.

Fitting should be assessed across the horizontal meridian.

The rule is to prevent excessive clearance (pooling) at the vertical meridian and excessive touch at the horizontal meridian (Figs 12.10A and B).

Fluorescein evaluation on astigmatic cornea

	Optimum	*Steep*	*Flat*
Central	Light touch	Pooling	Touch
Horizontal meridian (with the rule astigmatic cornea)	Mild touch	Touch in the vertical meridian	Excessive touch in the horizontal meridian
Edge width	Optimum	Narrow	Wide at vertical meridians

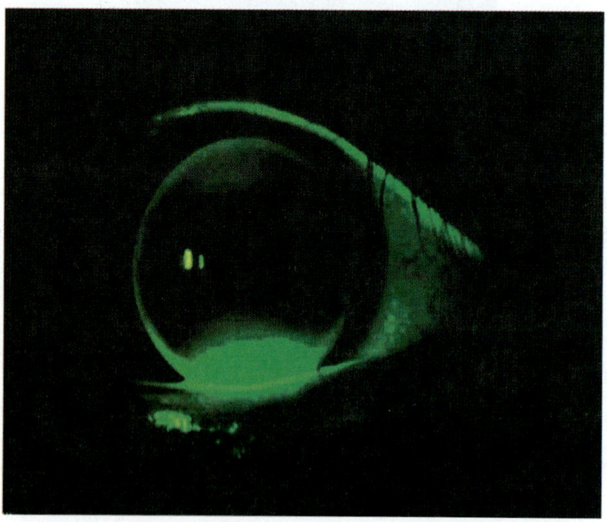

Fig. 12.10A: Spherical RGP on astigmatic cornea

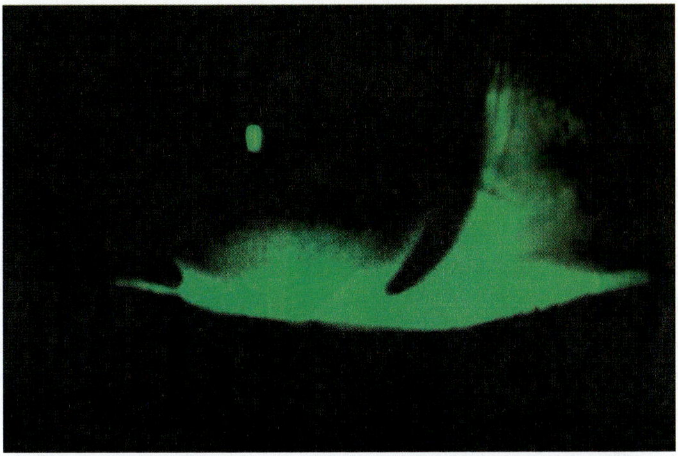

Fig. 12.10B: Spherical RGP on astigmatic cornea

Lens thickness and material flexibility influence the amount of astigmatism corrected.

Modifications/alterations on the basis of the fluorescein pattern observed

Central

Pooling / clearance	Flatten base curve
Touch / bearing	Steepen base curve

Mid-peripheral

Touch	Flatten base curve	Reduce diameter	Flatten peripheral curves
Pooling	Steepen base curve	Increase diameter	Steepen peripheral curves

Edge

If central fit steep and narrow edge	Flatten base curve
If central fit flat and wide edge	Steepen base curve
If good central fit and narrow edge	Wide edge—Flatten PC/ increase PC width Steepen PC/decrease PC width

Diameter

Altering the diameter is done on the basis of the corneal and the pupil coverage. Remember *if the diameter is increased the lens will behave steep or tight.* Suitable adjustments have to be made to the base curve if the diameter is increased or decreased. Diameter modifications also help if:

Lens rides high and does not drop with blink—Reduce diameter

Lens rides low or shows rapid drop after blink —Increase diameter

Lens positions continually to one side—Increase diameter

Once the base curve , diameter, peripheral curves are decided the next step is over refraction.

Over Refraction

With the trial lens on the eye the procedure of retinoscopy and acceptance is done. This is done to:

- calculate the tear lens power and compensate for it
- calculate the residual astigmatism, if any
- recheck the best visual acuity, cross checks if any errors are made in spectacle corrections
- Reconfirm, if the fitting is proper. An improper fitting will result in unstable and fluctuating vision
- Any flexure problems.

Following are some examples of final lens power based on fitting relationship and over refraction.

The calculations are based on the tear lens phenomenon. A steep lens will create a positive tear lens so minus power of same amount has to be added to compensate for it and the flat lens will create a negative tear lens so plus power has to be added.

Power calculation and tear lens (examples)

Contact lens power as calculated from spectacle Rx	*Trial lens power*	*Fitting relationship*	*Over refraction*	*Final power of the contact lens to be ordered*
–2.50	–3.0	Alignment	+0.50	–2.50
–2.50	–3.0	Steep by 0.05 mm (0.25D)	+0.25 (–0.25 for tear lens)	–2.75
–2.50	–3.0	Flat by 0.05 mm (0.25 D)	+0.75 (+0.25 D for the tear lens)	–2.25

Central Thickness and Flexure and the Material to be Ordered

It is best to select a lens material with highest Dk available for the benefit of the patient. Each RGP material has its critical thickness. If made thinner than that, the phenomenon of flexure will happen on the eye. Flexure leads to unwanted induced astigmatism and unstable vision. The central thickness of the lens depends upon the power of the lens to be ordered.

Tint

Any light shade tint is can be ordered for the lens. This tint does not change the eye color but is only for easy handling and identification in the container. This is actually impregnated in the button during polymerization.

The final order of an RGP lens includes

1. BC
2. Power
3. OD
4. OZ

5. IC/width
6. PC/width
7. C Th
8. Tint
9. Material.

SUMMARY: STEPS

1. Refraction
2. Keratometry
3. Eye examination
4. Other eye parameters
5. Select the trial lens
6. Assess fit
   - *Dynamic*
   - *Static fitting*
7. Finalize the curvatures and diameter
8. Over refraction
9. Order.

13 Soft Toric Contact Lens Fitting

Soft toric contact lens fitting for astigmatic eyes is supposed to be a specialty fitting, whereas the modern designs and fitting guidelines have simplified so much that they are as easy as a spherical soft lens fitting. An additional understanding of the design, its axis and power calculation is needed to fit an astigmatic eye.

Astigmatic correction upto 4 .0 diopters can be achieved with rigid spherical lenses. With spherical soft lenses spectacle cylinder is acceptable upto 0.75 diopter can only be corrected. The incidence of astigmatism surveys that 16% of prescriptions have more than 1.0 diopter of astigmatism, which increases to 30% with 0.75D or more of astigmatism.

With the increasing demand for comfort and better visual acuity soft toric lenses are getting popular now.

We have various options to correct astigmatic eyes like

1. Spherical RGP
2. Toric RGP (not available in India)
3. Soft toric lenses.

Indications for Prescribing Soft Toric Contact Lens (Fig. 13.1)

1. When the best sphere (spherical equivalent) does not give a satisfactory visual acuity.
2. When there is residual astigmatism more than 0.75 diopters with spherical soft lenses. This residual cylinder causes discomfort/asthenopia to the wearer.

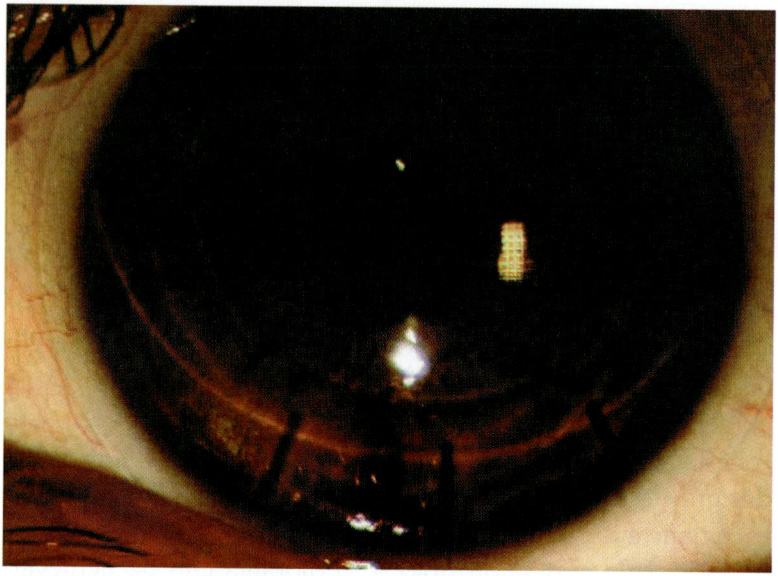

Fig. 13.1: A soft toric lens

3. When the rigid gas permeable lens is uncomfortable.
4. When the **sphere to cylinder ratio is less than 4:1.**

Spectacle refraction	*Ratio Sph : cyl*	*Toric CL indicated?*
– 3.0 Ds / – 0.75 Dc	3 : 0.75	Not necessary
– 8.0 Ds /– 1.50 Dc	4 : 0.75	Not necessary
– 0.50 Ds /– 1.0 Dc	4 : 8	Yes
– 12 .0 /– 2.0 Dc	4 : 0. 75	Not necessary

5. It depends on patients' visual needs. Some may be satisfied with the visual acuity, which may not reach the 6/6 target with spherical lenses, and some may be very sensitive about the sharpness of visual acuity.
6. Uncorrected astigmatism can be tolerated in non-dominant eye but not in the dominant eye.
7. A spherical refraction with corneal astigmatism does not need a toric contact lens.

Since, soft toric lenses available in our country this chapter will discuss the fitting philosophies of soft toric lenses only.

A spherical soft lens has only one curvature whereas a toric lens has two different radii of curvature in two principal meridians. In case of toric spectacle lenses we order the cylindrical axis and the fitter fits it in the spectacles according to the axis specified. This does not happen in the eye. The lens rotates and behaves different in every eye. This is due to different anatomy and lid positions of an individual eye.

So, all soft toric lenses have a stabilization technique to prevent axis mislocation on the eye.

The lids and the lid forces hold the contact lens in the palpebral space. Lens movement will attempt to move the lens in the same direction as itself. In case of toric lens, the rotational movement is made stable in the vertical axis.

Good vision with any kind of toric lens needs stable cylinder axis location.

The soft toric lenses **stabilizing mechanisms** are (Fig. 13.2):

- Prism ballast
- Truncation
- Peri-ballast
- Double slab-off
- Reverse prism

Prism Ballast

In this technique 1 to 1.5 D base down prism is incorporated near the inferior periphery of a round lens. The prism acts as a weight and prevents rotation. The stability is thus provided by the difference in thickness. Based on the watermelon seed principle the thin edge of the round lens lies under the upper lid and the thicker edge rests over the lower lid. This is the simplest and most common adapted technique for stabilization of a toric lens.

This design creates some discomfort along the lower lid margin due to thick edge. This thick edge also reduces the oxygen transmissibility at the lower thick edge of the lens.

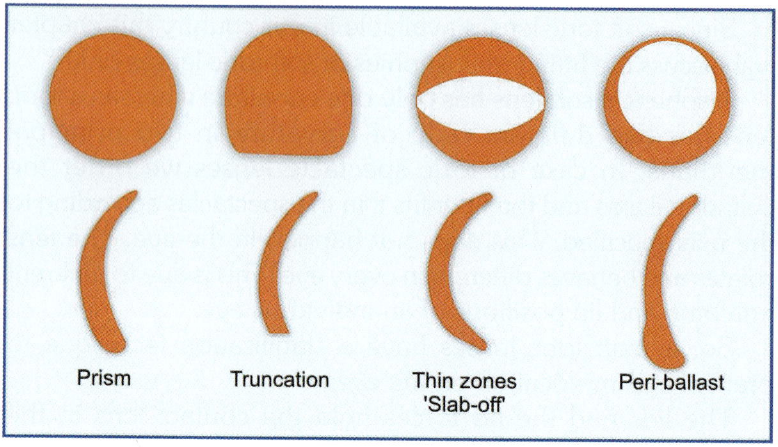

Fig. 13.2: Toric designs

Truncation

In this technique the lower portion of the lens is cut horizontally, so that the lens rests on the lower lid and is stabilized. These truncated edges may be source of discomfort. This technique is also not always successful in practice as truncation alters the thickness profiles and differentials. It is also difficult to manufacture and finish (Fig. 13.3).

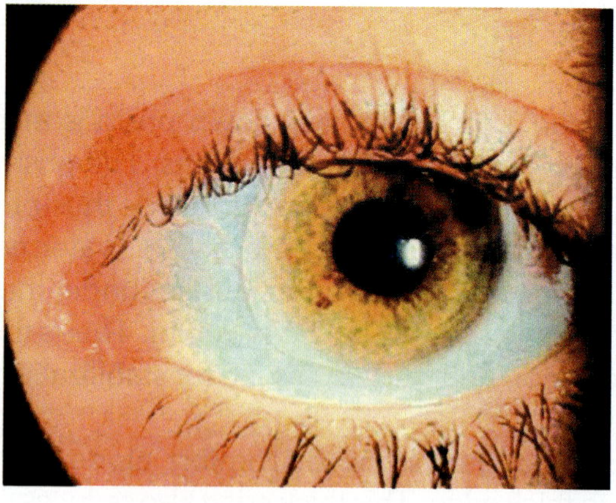

Fig. 13.3: Truncated lens

Peri-ballast

This technique utilizes the minus carrier design at the edge. This is then converted to create a prism base down effect and uses the thickness differences as stabilizing component.

This technique like prism ballast may cause discomfort at the lower lid and reduce oxygen transmissibility at the thicker edge.

Double Slab-off

Thin zones are first created at the edges. Due to lid interaction and thickness profile the lenses are stabilized. The thin zones upper and lower interact with the lids especially the upper lid, to position and stabilize the lens on the eye.

This lens has better comfort due to reduced lens thickness. This design may not work in patients with loose lids.

Reverse Prism Designs

This design incorporates two prisms one base up and other base down prism. Chamfering is done at the prism base to cut off the inferior edge horizontally which reduces the discomfort and creates a prism less optic zone.

It is an advancement of the prism ballast design.

Based on the surface where the cylindrical power is the toric lens is classified below.

Types of Toric Lenses

- Back toric
- Front toric
- Bitoric

Front Surface Toric

When the front surface has two radii of curvature and the back surface is spherical. This corrects total refractive astigmatism.

Back Surface Toric

The (base curve) posterior curve has two different radii of curvature at two principal meridians and the front surface is spherical. These lenses will correct the corneal astigmatism.

Bitoric

Both anterior and posterior surfaces have two different radii of curvature at two principal meridians. These lenses also correct the total refractive astigmatism. These lenses are also uncommon.

Axis Marks on Toric Soft Lens

Some form of reference mark is needed on the toric lens to assess the rotation. Different manufacturers have different markings. They may be permanent (usually) a laser or mechanical engraving or a temporary one with an ink or dye. They are either a single or 3 marks with a specific separation angle at the 6 o'clock or horizontal axis. One must refer to manufacturer's guidelines before estimating rotation.

Lens markings are for reference only (Fig. 13.4).

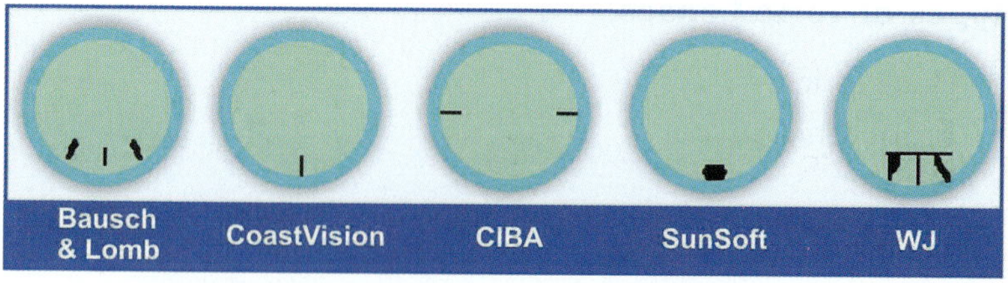

Fig. 13.4: Lens markings (various manufacturers)

Fitting Guidelines

Step 1

Perform refraction. (minus cylinder form). Be very accurate.

Step 2

Do keratometry.

Step 3

Estimate the total astigmatism.
Total astigmatism = corneal astigmatism + internal astigmatism

Step 4

Selection of the trial lens:
Select the design on the basis of the type of astigmatism.

Base Curve and Diameter

Select the base curve as per the keratometry and the diameter on the basis of HVID. The selection is made the same way as in the spherical soft lens.

Power and Axis

The trial set consists of two axis 180 and 90 degrees in the base curves available. Select the lens, the axis of the cylinder, which is closest to spectacle prescription. *If the minus cylinder axis is near 180 degrees select the 180 degree reference lens, and if the minus cylinder axis is near 90 degrees select the 90 degree axis reference trial lens.*

The power of the trial lens is immaterial. The purpose of the trial lens is to calculate the axis rotation.

The power of the contact lens is calculated from the spectacle prescription. *Over refraction is not performed in finalizing the power of the lens.*

Disposable Toric Contact Lens

The method is to order a trial lens based on empirical calculations from the spectacle prescription and keratometry. The final orders are made with adjustments, if needed, on this lens.

Step 5

Insert the trial lens and wait for 15 to 20 minutes.

Step 6

Evaluate physical fit and measurement of lens rotation.
Physical fit – finalize the base curve first.

Finalize the base curve first the same way as spherical soft lens (Fig. 13.5).

Calculate the rotation as explained in the next step, on the base curve and diameter, which will be ordered in the final. Do not calculate the rotation if any unless the BC and OD are finalized.

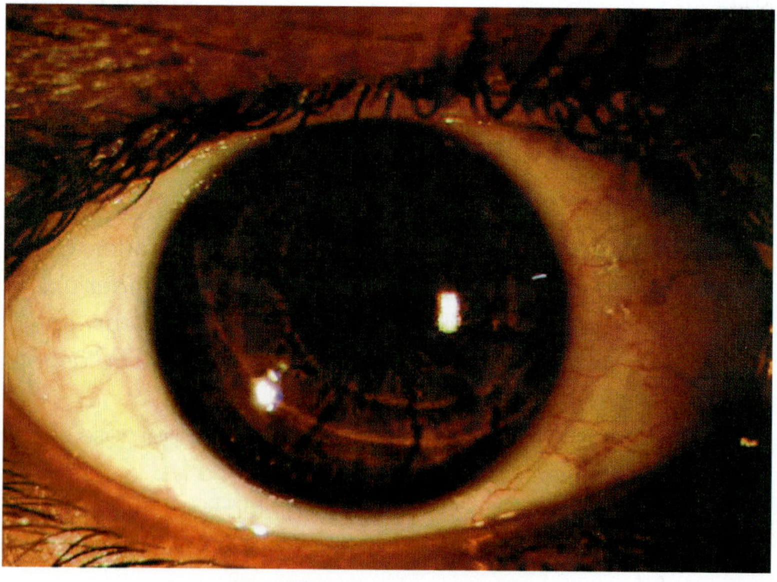

Fig. 13.5: Assess soft fit first

Measurement of Lens Rotation

The rule is based on the principle of LARS or CAAS

To identify the lens rotation, observe the markings on the lens. (Depends on the manufacturer)

Suppose, the trial lens has 3 orientation markings at 5, 6, 7 o' clock position of the lens. The separation of each marking is 30 degrees (one clock hour is equal to 30 degrees). The position of the lens if shifts such that the 5 o'clock marking shifts to 6 o'clock position the lens is supposed to have rotated by 30 degrees (Fig. 13.6).

If the lens rotates to the practitioner right (anticlockwise) subtract that many degrees from the axis of the spectacle prescription. If it rotates to practitioner left (clockwise) add that many degrees of rotation to the spectacle prescription.

L	A	R	S
Left	Add	Right	Subtract

Note

1. *Add or subtract from the spectacle axis prescription.*
2. *Left means practitioners' left.*

Suppose the spectacle prescription is: – 2.0 Dsph / –2. 25 D cyl × 180.

If the rotation of the lens is 10 degrees to the left—the axis ordered will be

10 degrees left – 2.0 Ds / – 2. 25 × 180
add 10

– 2.00/ – 2.25 × 10

If the rotation is 10 degrees to right then the final axis to be ordered is

10 degrees right – 2.0 / – 2.25 × 180
Subtract 10

– 2.0 Ds / – 2.25 × 170

This compensation is made because—The refraction of the eye is – 2.0 / – 2.25 × 180. If the lens rotates by 10 degrees clockwise (left) when placed on the eye, the correction will now be – 2.0 / – 2.25 × 170. This will blur the vision. To compensate for this, if the lens ordered is – 2.0 / – 2.25 × 10, the 10 degree rotation will bring the axis to 180 degrees, which is required.

Note

- *The final lens will show the same degree of rotation when placed on the same eye (Fig. 13.7).*

Methods of measurement of rotation

i. Narrow slit beam of the slit-lamp (Fig. 13.8)
ii. Cylinder marking in the trial frame
iii. Protractor scale of the eye piece graticule
iv. Estimation from markings position (Fig. 13.9).

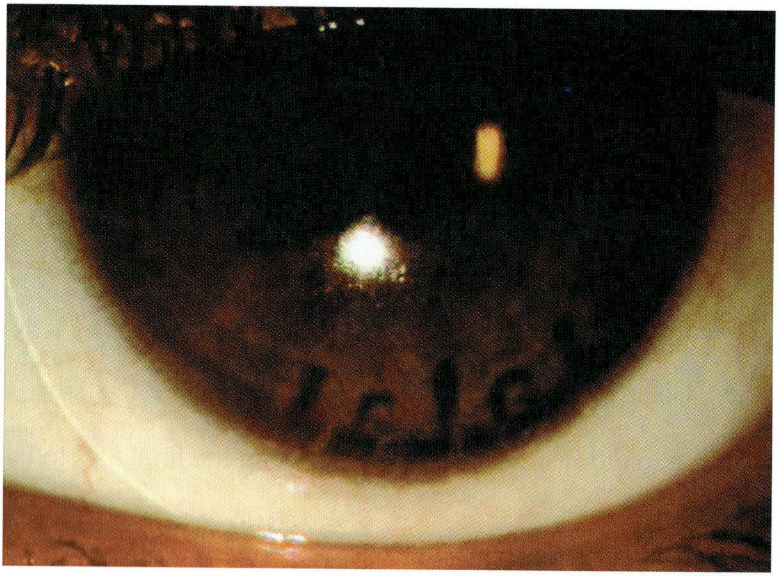

Fig. 13.6: Rotation to right

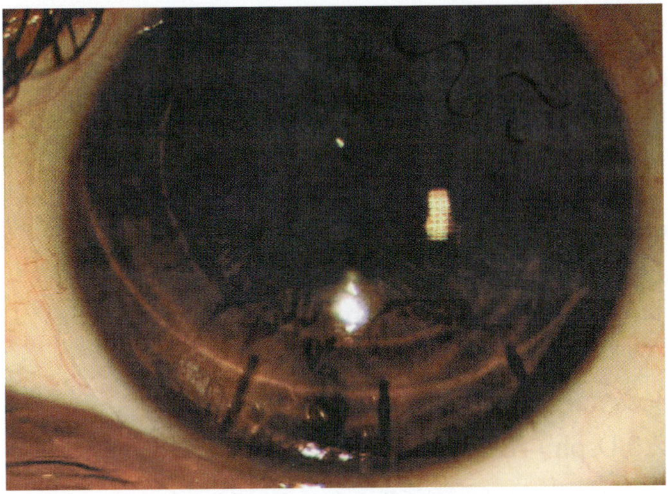

Fig. 13.7: Final lens markings will show same rotation as in trial

The axis rotation gives the practitioner the information needed to order the next lens. The rotation shows that how far the axis of the cylinder will be mislocated when the final lens will be placed on the eye.

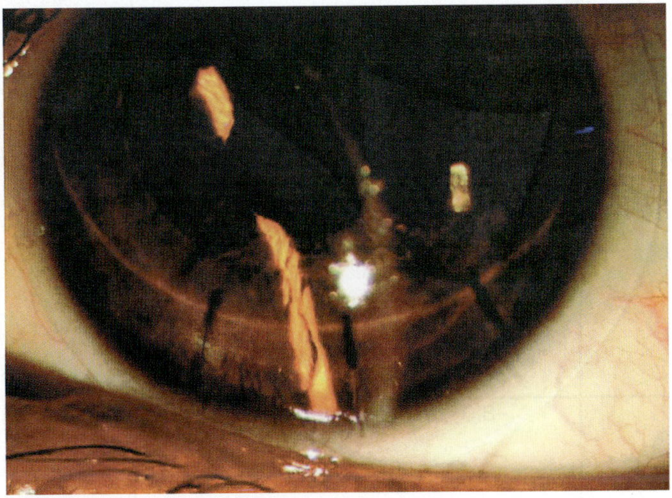

Fig. 13.8: Lens rotation calculation with slit

Step 7

Calculate the power from the spherical and the cylindrical from the spectacle prescription order power based on these calculation.

This calculation is done in following steps:

1. Writing the spectacle prescription in the cross cylinder form (at 2 principal meridians)
2. Then compensate for the back vertex
3. Rewrite in sphero cylinder form.

Suppose the spectacle power is

–2.0 Dsph / –3.0 cyl × 180

Write in principle meridian form and back vertex power

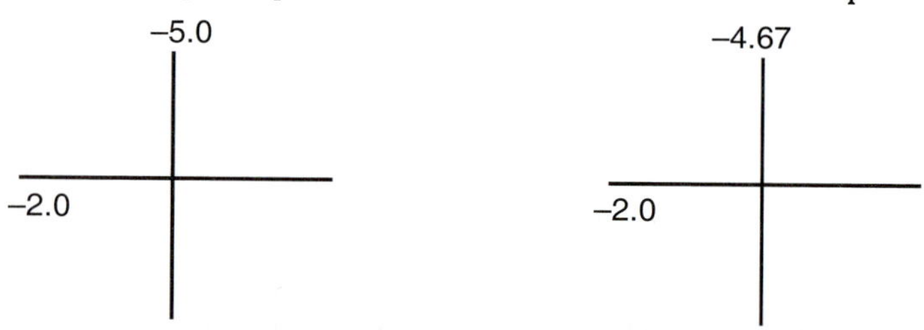

Rewrite in spherocylinder form (compensating BVP)= –2.0 Dsph / –2.67 d cyl × 180

Hence the power of the toric CL ordered is –2.0 Ds / –2.67 Dc × 180. (Take the cylinder value closest to the one available).

Taking one more example

–6.0 Dsph / –2.0 Dcyl × 90

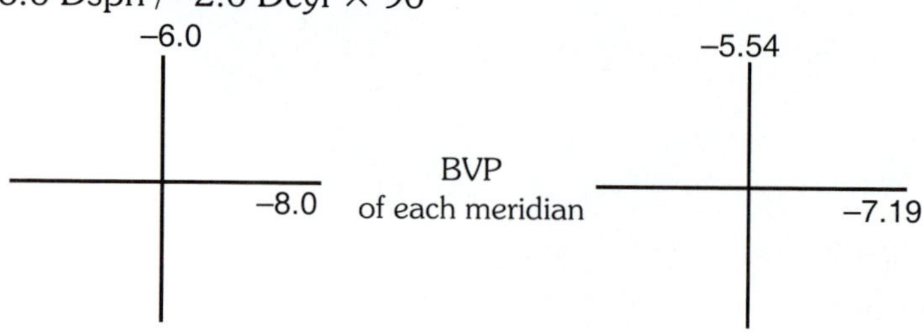

–5.54 Ds/ –1.65 Dcyl × 90

Step 8

Final order

- Base curve
- Power and axis
- Diameter
- Lens type (design)

Troubleshooting—Soft Toric Contact lenses

Poor vision It is the most common problem encountered. Most often the mistake is in:

- Axis mislocation
- Wrong power calculation
- Stabilization ineffectiveness of some designs.

If one encounters poor visual acuity

Step 1

Check, Is the lens rotationally stable on the eye?

Yes And the lens is orienting correctly

- Then check spectacle prescription
- Or check lens prescription.

No And the lens is rotating on the eye

- Which direction is it rotating—Clockwise/ anti-clockwise (Add or subtract)
- Alter lens fit—Base curve
- Change either the design or lens type.

Poor Comfort is mainly due to poor fitting

- Change the design
- Change the base curve.

Edema

- Poor transmissibility due to thick edge
- Thin mid water content dynamic stabilization better transmissibility.

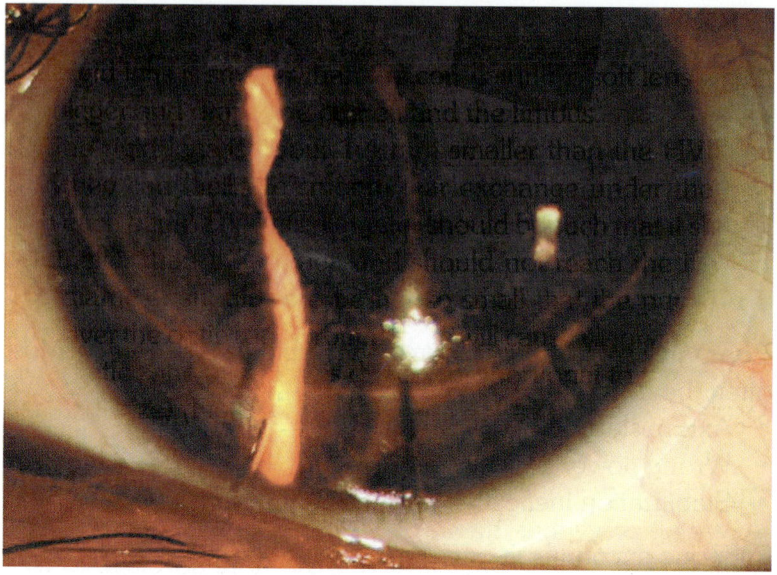

Fig. 13.9: Calculating rotation from markings position

Staining

- Possible due to less movement and tear exchange and entrapment of debris under the lens.

SUMMARY—TORIC SOFT LENS FITTING

1. Refraction—minus cylinder form
2. Keratometry
3. Eye examination and screening
4. Select the trial lens
   - Base curve on the basis of keratometry
   - Axis—180 or 90 on the basis of spectacle refraction
5. Assess fitting after stabilization
   - Finalize base curve and stabilization design
   - Calculate axis rotation—LARS rule
6. Calculate power
7. Compensate for axis rotation in the final power prescription.

14 Fitting Young Children with Contact Lens

Children are different from adults because they have different ocular surface, configuration and different physiology which is needed for the contact lens fitting.

Secondly children do not allow all the parameters and the trials to be done on the eye as easily as adults.

We all know that the reasons of fitting contact lens are not cosmetic. The basic principle is to allow more normal development of Visual Acuity and prevent or minimize amblyopia.

The reasons to prescribe contact lenses in children < 5 years are:

- High myopia
- Moderate to high hyperopia,
- Moderate to high anisometropia
- Amblyopia
- Nystagmus
- Corneal masking
- Bandage contact lens.

Children are fitted with contact lenses in moderate to high degrees of refractive error for simple reason that **contact lenses have following advantages over spectacles:**

- Reduce peripheral distortions
- Reduce aniseikonia
- Reduce prismatic imbalance
- Inappropriate correction in spectacles may interfere with emmetropization

- Better control in Eso deviations with contact lenses due to base out prism effect.

Contact Lens in Aphakic Child

This forms the largest part of pediatric Contact Lens Practice. We all know that favorable prognosis depends on surgical, optical correction followed by amblyopia therapy. CL reduces image size to 8% compared to 33% with glasses. This forms the major reason to fit lenses in this group. The aphakic spectacles are usually around +20 diopters in power, which make the glasses very heavy and unsightly.

Indication in Amblyopia

Occlusion contact lens is very useful for children who resist occlusion over spectacles with patches or occluder. Special contact lens with center opaque pupil and dark iris contact lenses are very easily acceptable to the parents also. One has to overrule the advantage over the risk of infections with the lenses. Second problem is that it has been seen that children can manipulate lens off cornea by rubbing the eyes. The major decision has to be from parents, who have to learn lens handling.

Cosmetic CL in Children

Cosmetic reasons to fit lenses in children are

- To mask opaque corneas
- Use in severe photophobia
- Aniridia, albinism, etc.

  Remember the advantages have to overrule risks.

Contact Lens in Nystagmus

Contact lens moves with visual axis so there are less distortions and prismatic effects, which will reduce the amplitude of nystagmus and hence better visual development.

As Bandage Lens

Contact lenses in children have same therapeutic reasons as in adults that is mostly for healing of epithelial aberrations as in trauma. It is very rare to find pediatric dystrophies and corneal syndromes.

Ocular Configuration Changes in Childhood

Compared to adults the child has following ocular change:

1. Have less *lipid deposits*
2. *Have increased aqueous*—hence good oxygen supply and maintains lubrication
3. Smaller *palpebral aperture* which inhibits insertion and removal.
4. Crying may lead to still tight closure of lids.

Pediatric Cornea

Before fitting lenses one must know the corneal dimensions in a child as this forms the basis of contact lens curvatures. These changes may affect the fit.

Corneal Diameter Changes in Childhood

The cornea in a child increases rapidly in first year of life and slowly thereafter.

- It is about 10 mm at birth
- About 11.5 mm at 4 years of age
- In microcornea and microphthalmia – diameter may range from 6 to 7 mm
- In megalocornea and high myopia diameter may range from 14 to 15 mm.

Corneal Curvature Changes in Childhood

- At birth about 47 to 49 D
- Rapid flattening in the first 6 months
- It flattens to 43.5D by 4 years of age.

- During first year the peripheral cornea is steeper which gradually flattens with age and growth.

Lens Designs and Materials for Children

Children can be fitted with either of these material lenses.
- RGP
- Soft
- Silicone elastomer.

The choice should be to give a lens that provides sufficient oxygen suitable as extended wear, comfort and vision. The lens should also be easy to handle for the parents.

Soft Contact Lens

This lens material has an advantage that it is comfortable. The comfort of the lens keeps the child quiet and willing.

Soft lens material in children has the following disadvantages:
- Difficult handling and insertion because they are large in size for their small palpebral apertures.
- Prone to deposits—like all soft lenses
- Infection risk in extended wear
- Limited parameters are available in soft lenses for pediatric age group. Lathe cut lenses or custom designs have to be ordered for children.

Rigid Gas Permeable Lens

Rigid lens materials as far as possible should be the lens of choice, due to its basic advantage of sufficient oxygen transmissibility.
- Easier for parents to handle
- Wide range of parameter available
- Excellent oxygen permeability
- Well tolerated due to moist eye.

Rigid lens materials in children have following difficulties:
- They are difficult to fit as one needs to align the lens curvatures to the atypical corneas.

- There is initial discomfort, which may discourage the parents and scare the child.
- Since these lenses move freely on the eye there is a possibility of lens dislodgment with rubbing.
- There may be corneal insult due to rubbing and rough insertion of these lenses.

Silicone Elastomers

Only available for pediatric aphakes in this group is the B&L – (Silsoft lens). It has enormous oxygen permeability but tends to coat lipids easily. This material is the only safe extended wear lens for children.

Now continuous wear **silicone hydrogels** are also available, they work as very safe and best lenses, if the suitable parameters are available for the child's eye.

Fitting Technique

Fitting Under GA

GA is recommended by some practitioners as it facilitates easy measurements, but involves risks of GA. Fit assessment is also found to be inaccurate under GA because:

- Lid position and forces are different in prone position
- Lacrimation is absent
- Decreased IOP which may change corneal shape

  Use *it only when it is impossible.*

Six Steps to Fit Infants and Very Young Children

1. ***Examine the eye:*** To rule out that the eye is ready for CL
2. ***Determine parameters for CL:*** Based on the ocular configurations some possible selections can be made even if the ocular dimensions are not measurable.
   a. *Select a lens diameter*
      - Soft lens—12 to 13 mm
      - RGP lens—9 to 9.5 mm
      - Silicone elastomer—11.3 mm

b. *Select a base curve*
   - Soft / silicone—one step steeper than the usual adult lens
   - RGP—0.10 to 0.20 mm steeper than usual.

c. *Central thickness:* Standard to thick, thin lenses should be avoided.

d. *Lens power:* The power of the lens should be ordered about 2- 3 diopters over plus than the spectacle refraction.

   The starting powers in aphakic according to age are usually found to be:

   6 months = +30
   1 year = +27
   2 years = +23
   3 years = +21

4. **Evaluation:** Evaluate the lens fit by checking the position and **movement** of lens. Wrap the infant properly in the sheet and hold him comfortable over the bed or mother's lap. Crying or squeezing will not allow you to assess the fit. Be calm and try to evaluate with the baby distracted or attracted by parents or relatives.

   In case of *Soft and Silicone lens*
   - Central position
   - Movement less than adults
   - Lens should not decenter more with blink and push up test.

   Fitting evaluation in RGP lens
   - Check position with torch and white light
   - Evaluate fluorescein pattern, with direct ophthalmoscope and blue filter
   - Prefer lid attachment fit

5. **Determine the final lens power:** After finalizing base curve and diameter do over refraction. Overplus infants by 2.5 to 3 D to give them the near working distance.

6. **Finalize:** See that the lens is stable on eye. Visibility or handling tint should be used. Ultimately again check that you prescribe a lens with sufficient oxygen to allow safe napping.

Instruction and Follow-up

Communication with parents is critical. Explain the risks and warning signs and the expenses. Reinforce that their efforts will make the child see better all life. This will encourage them to bear up with the shortcomings.

- **Insertion/removal**—both parents should be instructed (Fig. 14.1):
  - Restraint technique—Hold the child arms above head close to the skull therefore immobilizing the head and arm movements. The second person holds the legs together.
  - Straddling technique—the baby is swathed in thick blanket from neck downwards enveloping the rest of the body.

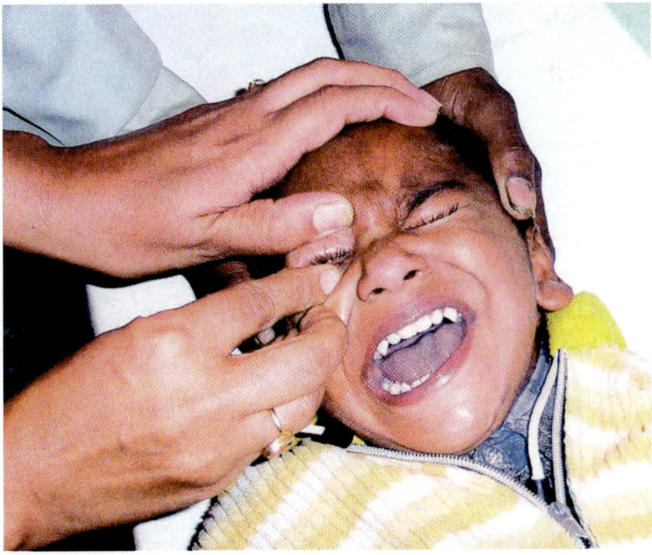

Fig. 14.1: Inserting an RGP lens

Follow-up

Children need to be followed up frequently, (monthly, 3 monthly) on every visit check:

- Compliance
- Over refraction
- Visual acuity—Teller's or HTOV charts
- Evaluate lens fit changes—this happens often as the cornea and the ocular dimensions are changing rapidly, especially in early years of life.

Remember the child's eye needs sufficient oxygen. The child is active so one has to fit a lens with more stable position, a lens that is more durable and easy to handle.

15 Fitting Contact Lenses in Presbyopes

In a survey, out of the population of people who need visual correction 27 percent are myopic and about 22 percent are presbyopic. This means that a large percentage of population needs correction for its presbyopia.

There are about 100 million presbyopes in India and 10 million are adding every year.

There are several options from spectacles to surgery, but our patients who started wearing lenses 15 to 20 years back are now turning presbyopic. It is usually, not acceptable to them to wear reading glasses over contact lenses. With the present trend, the presbyope now is leading an active life-style and has high disposable income. So it is expected that this group will form a large base in future contact lens practice.

Presbyopia

Presbyopia is part of the normal aging process, where the eye loses its ability to easily focus on near objects. Emmetropes, who have never worn glasses, will also require plus power to focus on near objects one has to just "Add" plus power to the patient's distance prescription to provide a lens that can focus on the near objects. We all know that presbyopia can be corrected by several options in spectacle form it can be by:

- Single vision reading glasses, bifocals, trifocals or multifocals

With contact lenses on the eye there are two options to correct near vision with spectacles over CL.

Option 1 is:

- Fit CL for distance; do not overcorrect

- Determine near addition over CL on trial frame
- Prescribe reading glasses over CL.

Option 2 is:
- Ideal for patients who do near/intermediate work all day
- Give near add on CL
- Give minus power for distance in the form of spectacles for driving and other distance task.

Patient Selection

Screening the patients is the key to success. Those who *are likely to respond positively* to presbyopic correction with contact lenses are the ones who are:
- Highly motivated
- Those who have adequate tear film and no lid disease or abnormality
- Have low hyperopia
- Whose jobs do not require fine visual acuity
- Affordability.

Contact Lens Presbyopia Correction

Three main types of contact lens for the presbyopic correction are:
- Monovision correction
- Alternating/translating vision lenses
- Simultaneous vision lenses.

Monovision (Fig. 15.1)

Monovision is the technique in which one eye is corrected for distance vision and the other eye for near vision. This is not occlusion. It works on the principle that the visual system can suppress the central focus image thus enable the object of interest to be seen clearly. There is some disruption of binocularity in this fitting methodology. Still Monovision remains the easiest

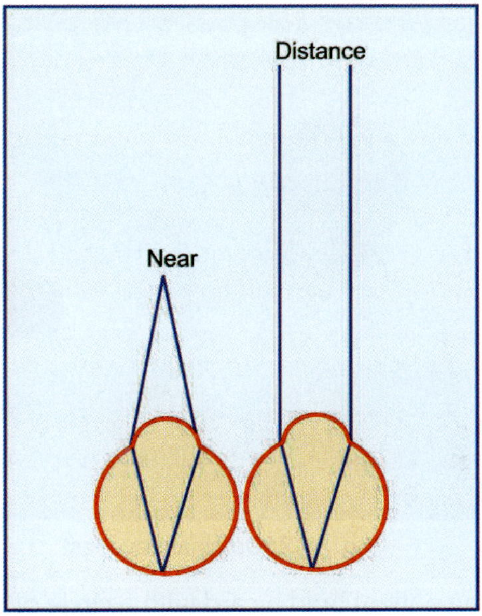

Fig. 15.1: Monovision: One eye corrected for near, other corrected for distance

and an effective means of correcting Presbyopia. The success rate is as high as 70%. This is the only technique by which we can correct the existing rigid lens wearers for near (as the options of bifocal RGP lenses are not yet available in our market). We can also convert emmetropes into contact lens wearers by simply fitting one eye for near.

Fitting Procedure for Monovision

1. Determine the distance and near prescription
2. Determine the **dominant and the non-dominant eye.** To do this, do the following test (Fig. 15.2):
   - Ask the patient to look at any distance object, may be a spot light or a bright colored dot target fixed at about 6 m distance or may be the 6/60 alphabet of the Snellen's chart.

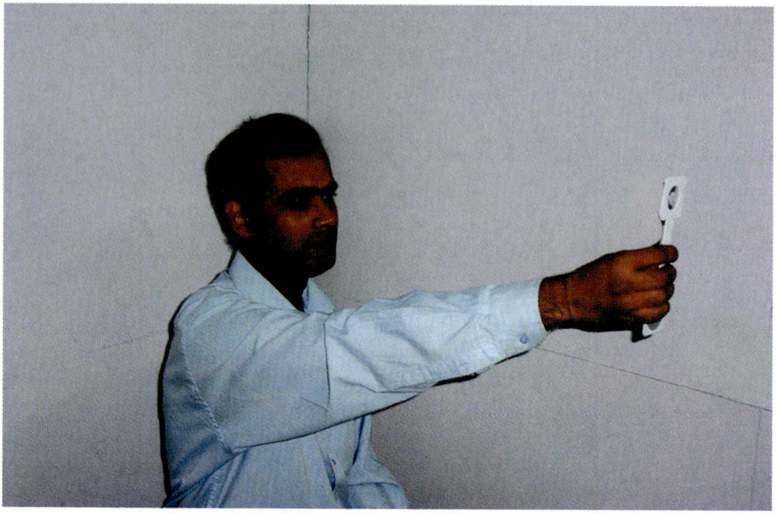

Fig. 15.2: Dominant eye test

- Let the patient hold a card with a circle of about 2 inches diameter at arms length
- Ask the patient to binocularly see through the circle, the distance spot light or any other target selected.
- Now alternately close his either eye. Ask through which eye, is he actually seeing the spot light.
- The patient will be able to see through one eye only. This is the dominant eye.

3. Fit the dominant eye with the distance power prescription and the non-dominant eye with the near power prescription. Suppose the patient's prescription is:
   RE : –4.0 Dsph and LE : –4.0 Dsph
   Near add +1.50 Dsph both eyes.
   Now fit the dominant eye with –4.0 Dsph (the distance power) and the non-dominant eye with –2.50 Dsph (the near power).
4. Use disposable lenses for this, and give an in-office trial. Record binocular visual acuity for distance and near. Most of them will be satisfied to see the magic of now being able to see for distance and near. Do not attempt uniocular visual

acuity now. Obviously the eye with near power will read less for distance and the eye with distance power will read less for near.

5. Explain the fitting technique now. Reassure that this will not harm his eyes.
6. Some patients may need some adaptation time and may be dissatisfied with the reduction of stereopsis.
7. Follow up, and fit the final lens.

Tips for Monovision fitting

- Adaptation time allowed should be at least 2 weeks
- Advise patients to continue normal activities if possible
- No night driving
- Do not compare eyes
- Set patient's expectations
- Educate visual improvement over time.

BIFOCAL/MULTIFOCAL CONTACT LENSES

Translating Vision Type (Fig. 15.3)

The patient must look and alternate through two separate portions to see either near or distant objects. This is just like our executive type bifocal spectacle lenses. The patient when looks down gaze the lower lid lifts the near segment up, towards the pupil or the visual axis thus the patient can see clear for near. This type of bifocal design is popular in rigid lens wearers. It needs a little more skill in fitting so that the position of the distance and the near segment is proper. In this design the near and far cannot be seen clearly at the same time. The fitting is assessed best with the Burton lamp than the slit lamp, so that it shows the position of the segments in more natural postures.

Advantages

- Sharp near/far vision
- When it works well, it is very successful
- Works better in RGP and less successful/common in SCL.

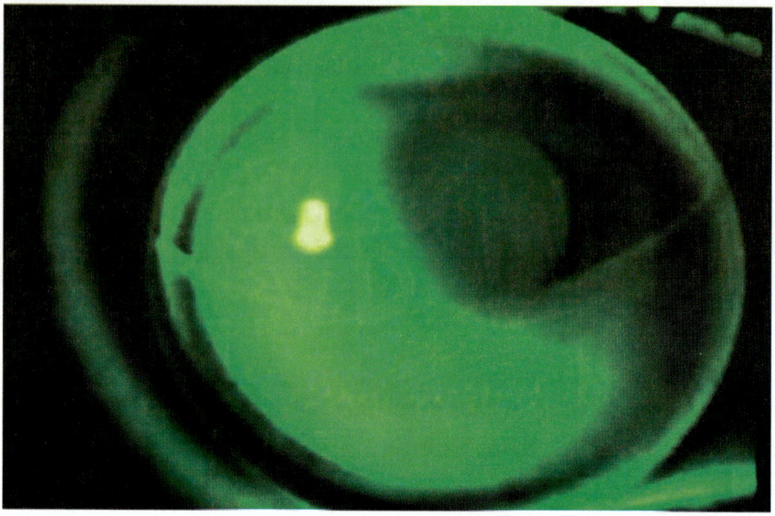

Fig. 15.3: Translating bifocal CL

Disadvantages

- Takes longer in adaptation
- Comfort is less due to thick design
- Dependence on eye-lens relationship.

Simultaneous Vision

In this type the distance and near images are focused on retina (fovea) simultaneously.

The brain will select or concentrate on one or other will be ignored. It is just like looking through the net across the window at a distance object. One must have noticed this that despite the net in the visual area the brain ignores it and you can see clear the distance target.

This technique may lead to "Ghosting" (doubling) of image, which may sometimes create a problem. Still it is the most popular option now in bifocal lenses.

Advantages

- Sharp near and far vision.

Disadvantages

- Compromised intermediate vision.
- Ghosting (doubling) is sometimes a problem.

Simultaneous vision lenses are further of three types:
- Concentric (segmented)
- Diffractive
- Aspheric.

Concentric Design

Concentric segment lenses show a sharp demarcation between distance and near powers.

They are of two types (Fig. 15.4):
- Center near
- Center distance

Central Near Segment

- Reading induced miosis, so it is good for patients who have more of near work to do
- In bright light the lens is biased for near.

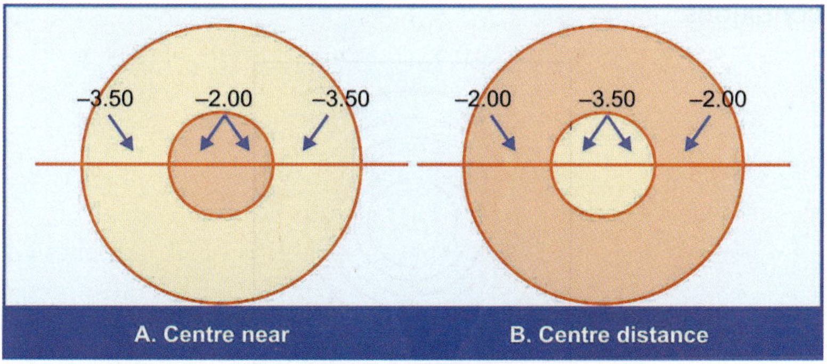

Fig. 15.4: Simultaneous bifocal: (A) Center near, and (B) Center distance

Central Distance Segment

- Pupil position is important in this design
- Halos may occur, if the pupil size exceeds the distance segment
- Interference from the segment images may be disturbing.

Pupil Size Dependency

There is dependency of these designs upon the pupil size. A center near will cause blurred vision for distance in bright light if the pupil constricts too low, and the distance center design can cause ghost images in night specially during driving.

Image clarity is relatively independent of pupil size like in multi-concentric design of Acuvue bifocal lens.

Diffractive Bifocal (Fig. 15.5)

Diffractive bifocal is made up of concentric rings, something like a Fresnel prism. Higher the addition more the number of rings.

- It has multiple circumferential Fresnel type prisms
- The distance and near images are focussed at the same time
- Pupil size is not important
- May not be good for excessive night driving
- Contrast sensitivity is reduced in this design.

It is most suitable for people who work in different light conditions.

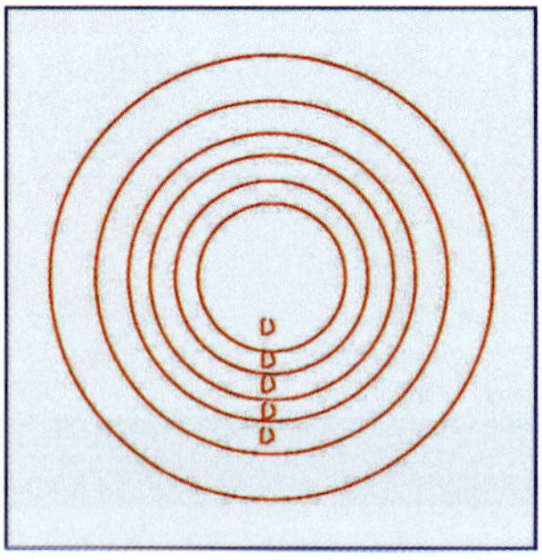

Fig. 15.5: Diffractive bifocal

Aspheric Designs (Fig. 15.6)

This is a progressive addition type of lens formed with alteration in anterior and posterior curvature of the lens. The power uniformly increases/ decreases in periphery due to the asphericity

- No ghosting as in concentric design
- Clarity of vision at all distances
- Simplified fitting
- Used mostly for office workers
- Disadvantage—pupil dependency.

It is of two types:

Aspheric back surface lens design

- Fit well over aspheric cornea
- Has Aspheric posterior curve
- Increasing PLUS power peripherally
- Provide central distance correction

Used in patients who need better distance vision in bright light.

Aspheric front surface lens design

- Aspheric anterior curve
- Back surface is spherical
- Increasing PLUS power centrally
- Provide central near correction.

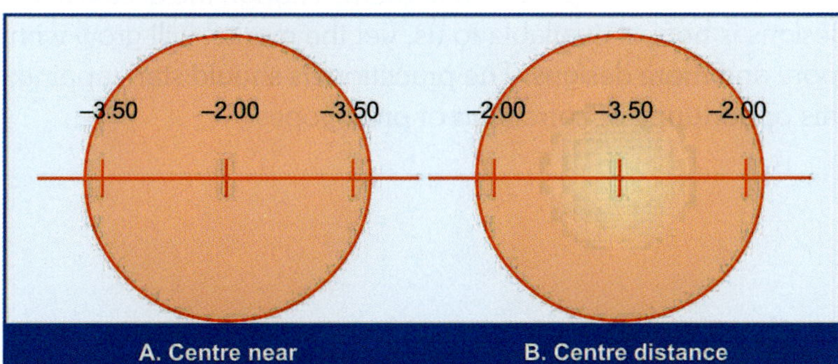

Fig. 15.6: Aspheric bifocal lens: (A) Center near and, (B) Center distance

Modified Monovision

This is a technique where one eye is fitted with distance correction and the other eye is a bifocal lens.

This improves the binocularity and stereoacuity which may be reduced in Monovision. This technique is also tried in patients who are sensitive to distance vision.

Unsuccessful contact lens fitting is likely in presbyopes who are:

- High myopes
- Patients with busy schedules
- Dry eyes
- Flat corneas
- Laxity of lower lid
- High astigmatism
- Or any other external ocular disease or abnormality.

SUMMARY

The number of patients who would require fitting of presbyopia is expected to increase in near future. The availability of single use of disposable lenses allows ease and trial for both patients and practitioners. *The fitting procedure is same and does not require extra skill to fit them.* One has to understand the design and the need of the patient to fit them. Though the access to all designs is not yet available to us, yet the market will grow with more and more designs. The practitioners should start tapping, this opportunity of correction of presbyopes.

16 Keratoconus

Keratoconus is a non-inflammatory degenerative abnormal condition of cornea which causes a conic deformity. It is usually bilateral and progressive. The thinning is mostly central and makes the cornea steeper by several diopters. This condition begins at puberty and progresses with varying degrees in individuals usually till 40-45 years of age. The protrusion leads to high astigmatism, myopia and irregular astigmatism. Due to the irregular refraction through the eye, vision may not improve to pinhole vision with spectacles.

Rigid contact lens is the best method of visual correction.

Early Detection of Keratoconus

Following are the signs which indicate keratoconus:

- Scissors retinoscopic reflex/oily droplet reflex
- Irregular, malapposed, malaligned, malshaped, malfocused pulsating keratometry mires
- Usually steep corneal curvature readings on keratometry
- Vision not improving to 6/6 with spectacles
- Rapidly increasing myopia and astigmatism
- Frequent change in glasses
- Polyopia
- Thinning of cornea on slit lamp and on pachymetry.

Keratoconus starts with irregular reflex and progresses to pronounced conical cornea and later advances to scarring and hydrops of the cornea. The advanced stages may need corneal transplantation (Fig. 16.1).

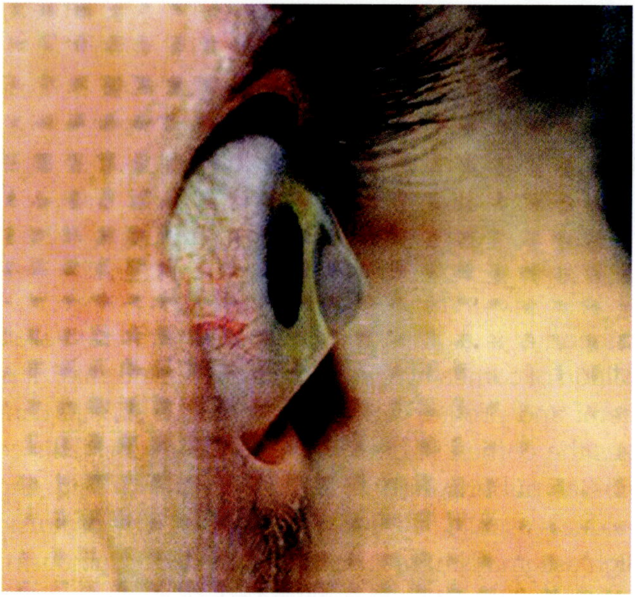

Fig. 16.1: Keratoconus

Keratoconus can be classified into three types on the basis of the cone shape:

1. Nipple type—is most common, and easy to fit lenses
2. Oval type—is usually sagging and difficult to fit
3. Globus cone—much larger and involves large corneal area.

CORRECTION OF KERATOCONUS WITH CONTACT LENSES

The contact lens works well in improving visual acuity by correcting the irregular astigmatism and retrieving the shape of the disordered anterior surface.

It is not definite that contact lenses retard the progression of the keratoconus.

Several types of contact lens designs may be used in keratoconus:

- Bicurve/tricurve rigid gas permeable lenses
- Soper lenses

- Soft lenses
- Piggy back lenses
- Scleral lenses.

Keratometry Readings

Keratometry readings are distorted, malapposed, malaligned, malshaped, malfocused and pulsating. K readings may not be easily obtainable due to the distortion of the mires. However, an approximate reading can be taken. If possible one should get the topography done.

Keratoconus can be classified on the basis of K readings.

- < 45.0 D = mild
- > 45.0 D = moderate
- > 52.0 D = advanced
- > 60.0 D = severe

The range of the keratometer is upto 52.0 D which can be extended by holding +1.25 lens in front of the objective. The readings have then to be recalibrated from the table of extended range (9 Diopters, have to be approximately added to obtain the reading).

Fitting Technique

The trial method is the best and the only possible method of fitting contact lenses in keratoconus. One cannot empirically calculate the lens curvatures and power.

1. In case of very early keratoconus, soft lenses can be tried, provided the vision improves satisfactorily with them.
2. The second choice is the rigid spherical lens. This also works in early keratoconus.
3. Soper design is the choice in moderate to advanced cases
4. Piggy back or special designs like Rose K lenses can be tried in cases where the rest fail.

To start with the fitting steps:

1. **Do refraction** and record best corrected spectacle visual acuity. Though this will not match with the contact lens power in most of the cases.
2. Do **keratometry or topography** as far as possible.
3. Perform a slit lamp **anterior segment examination to** rule out any contraindication.
4. Select the trial lens from the special keratoconus trial set. - initial lens is flatter than the K.
5. Evaluate the **fluorescein pattern** to achieve the good fit, i.e. the **three point touch** (Fig. 16.2).
   - Central touch of 2-3 mm
   - Thin band of touch at lens periphery
   - Review the centration and the movement with the blink.
6. Exchange lenses until the light desirable apical touch is achieved.
7. Do **over refraction** and finalize the power.

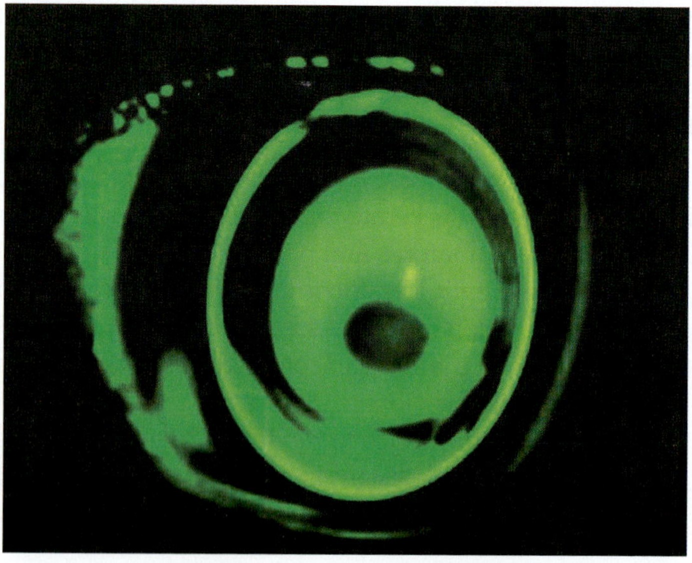

Fig. 16.2: Three point touch

Tips for Parameters Selection in Keratoconus

Diameter

The diameter of the keratoconus lenses ranges from 8.0 to 10.0 mm.

- Select larger diameters as far as possible—gives better stability, comfort and large optic zone for better vision
- Large diameters may not show good exchange in steep central nipple type of keratoconus. Select a smaller lens in that case 8.0 to 8.5 mm. This lens is usually bicurve and centering difficult to achieve at times.

Peripheral Curves

The lenses are tricurve or multicurve. Multicurve designs are needed to match the highly aspheric corneas. In keratoconus the cornea may show central reading ranging form 45 to 60 and the peripheral readings from 35 to 40 diopters. There is a great amount of aphericity found. A normal design lens will rock and show excessive edge lift. The added curves are made flatter and flatter to contour the peripheral shape of the cornea (Fig. 16.3).

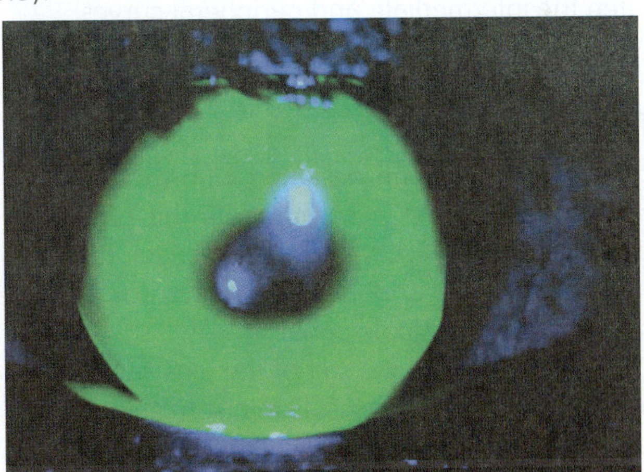

Fig. 16.3: Normal design lens will rock and show excessive edge lift

Power Calculation

The best way to determine power of the contact lens, is to do refraction over the trial lens, on the patient's eye. Finalize the fitting curvatures first and then do the over refraction. Just add algebraically the power in the trial lens and the over add. Compensate for back vertex power if needed. The powers are usually high minus. A properly fitted lens can give 6/6 vision with spherical power. If there is any residual cylindrical correction required, it can be added over the spectacles.

Suppose, the trial lens is 52.0/ –4.50/ 9.4 on the eye. An additional power of –3.0 diopters is needed over it to achieve 6/6. The final contact lens power to be made is –7.50 Ds. In case there is a residual cylinder, which cannot be compensated by the spherical equivalent, prescribe in spectacles over the glasses.

Judgment—During Fluorescein Evaluation

1. A bubble—flatten the base curve
2. Excessive apical touch—Steepen the base curve
3. Normal apical touch and excessive touch at the periphery – flatten the intermediate and peripheral curves
4. Fluctuating vision—reevaluate the fit.

Soper Lens Design

The Soper lens has been designed with a very steep central posterior base curve to accommodate the protrusion of the cornea. The peripheral curves are much flatter. It gives excellent results in moderate and advanced keratoconus patients, especially those with nipple cones.

The apical height or the sag of the lens can be made more by increasing the diameter just like in soft lenses.

Fitting

The lens trial set has certain series of lenses, which are designed for moderate, advanced and severe cases. Select the lens according to the severity and achieve.

- 2-3 mm apical touch
- Centration
- Movement

Piggy Back Lenses (Fig. 16.4)

It is the method of fitting a rigid lens over the soft lens. The soft forms a uniform base for the rigid lens to stabilize and provides comfort to the patient. This method should be tried in advanced cases when other method fails. This system also needs two types of lens care solutions and may cause handling problems. The soft lens usually 8.4 mm/14.0 mm is fitted on the eye. The rigid lens curve and power is calculated over it.

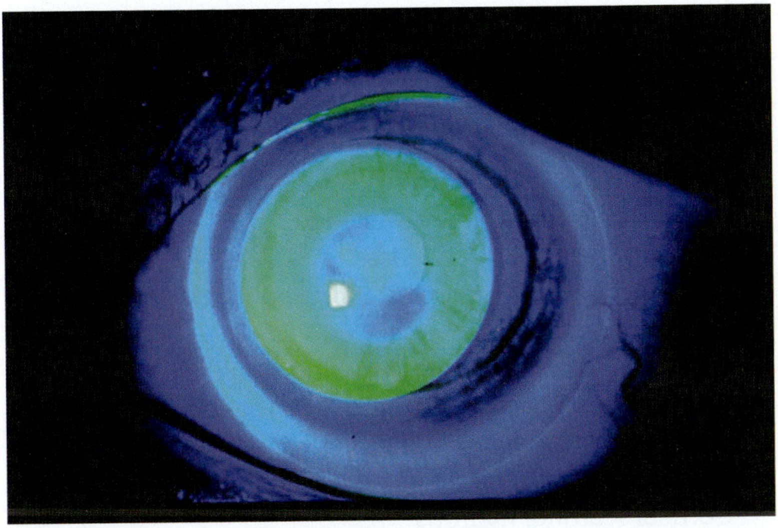

Fig. 16.4: Piggy back lens

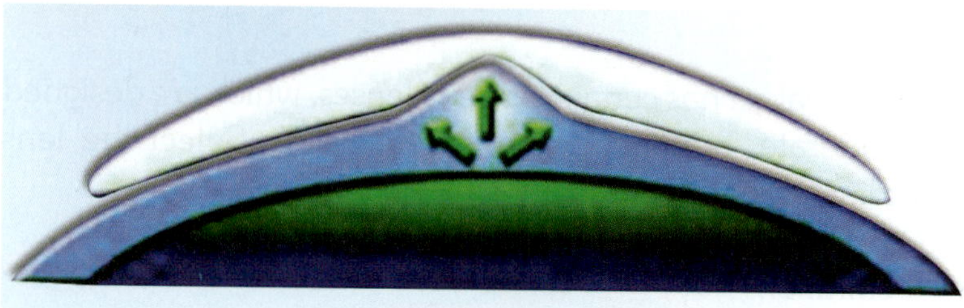

Fig. 16.5: Rose K lens

Rose K Lens (Fig. 16.5)

The Rose K lens is probably the most widely fitted keratoconus lens worldwide and achieves an 85% first fit success. The Rose K lens design is a fully flexible lens, with multiple parameters that works well on early to advanced keratoconus patients. Complex lens geometry, combined with the enhanced material benefits of Boston ES™, makes the Rose K lens the good fit enhancing patient comfort and visual acuity.

Progression

Keratoconus tends to progress, which leads to increasing myopia. With the increasing protrusion the lens apical touch may increase with time leading to complications and intolerance of lenses. These patients should be reviewed every 6 months, and refitted with new curvatures whenever needed.

Asking patient to be off lenses for at least 48 hours before refitting the patient. The topography should also be repeated and changes recorded.

Despite lenses, depending on an individual the keratoconus progresses. In severe cases the fitting of lenses becomes difficult. The patient should be considered for keratoplasty if

- The lenses cannot be tolerated for 10 hours
- Corneal scarring, hydrops
- Corneal thinning upto 0.3 mm
- Vision achieved with lenses is less than 6/18.

Fitting keratoconus patient's needs patience, as several lenses may need to be changed before a successful fit is achieved. It is finally very satisfying as these are the patients who will benefit from your skill, in achieving vision.

17 Therapeutic Contact Lenses

It is common to fit contact lenses for optical or cosmetic reasons, but contact lenses are also used for therapeutic purposes also, particularly in hospital based practice. Perhaps the first contact lens was fitted for therapeutic reasons rather than cosmetic.

With improvements in materials which transmit more oxygen, therapeutic lenses are finding wider applications as medical and surgical adjunct. *Contact lens practitioner need to work along with ophthalmologist to fit these lenses for the benefit of the patient.*

Even if the practitioner does not fit lenses for therapeutic purposes, still all should have a working knowledge of the conditions appropriate for the treatment or what to do with the existing therapeutic lens-wearing patient.

Therapeutic lenses are also called **bandage lenses** that are used to treat a range of external ocular surface disorders primarily affecting cornea.

The Therapeutic Lenses Principle Aim is to Bandage the Eye Serving as a Therapy which

- Provides relief from pain.
- Serves mechanical protection by separating the epithelial surface from the external agents such as lid surfaces, thus protecting the epithelium.
- Seal corneal perforations by acting as a splint for the underlying weaker tissues and supports the area while healing takes place.

- Corrects the surface irregularities in irregular corneas and improves visual acuity.

Unlike normal corneas the eye to be fitted with therapeutic lens is a compromised eye and is at higher risk of hypoxia and infections. The balance between benefits and potential risk must be carefully considered.

Conditions of Eye which are Suitable for Therapeutic Lenses

1. Eyelid abnormalities—entropion, trichiasis, ectropion, lagophthalmos
2. Ocular surface disorders—chemical injuries, dry eye, Stevens-Johnson syndrome
3. Corneal surface disorder—recurrent erosion syndrome, keratitis, traumatic epithelium abnormalities, filamentary keratitis, bullous keratopathy.

Lens materials that can be used as extended wear are:

1. Hydrogels
2. Silicone hydrogels
3. High Dk RGP lenses
4. Collagen shields
5. Scleral lenses.

Hydrogels—Soft Lenses

HEMA lenses used for extended period are a choice dependent on the corneal pathology.

i. *High water content soft lenses:* Lenses with water content 80% and Plano power are available as bandage lens. They are suitable for epithelial defect patients. These lenses act as bandage which necessitate minimal epithelial disturbance and help in relieving pain (Fig. 17.1).

ii. *Mid water content lenses:* Lenses with 45 to 60% water content may be the choice for small perforations or leaking wounds. They act as a splint.

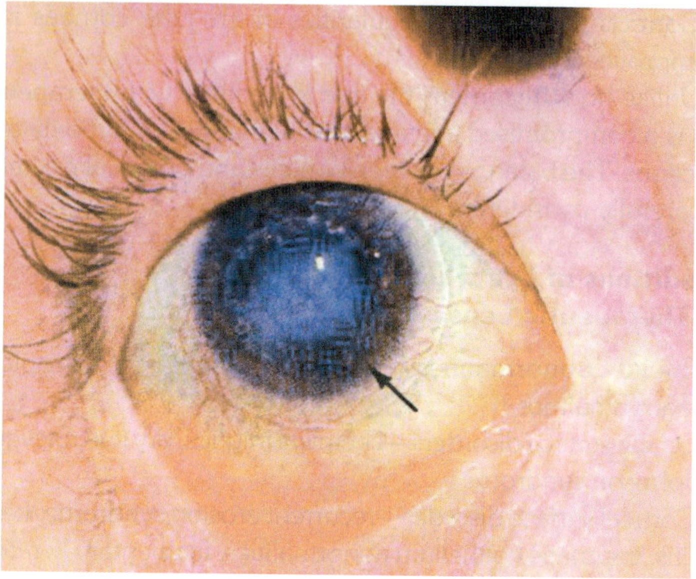

Fig. 17.1: Soft lens as bandage lens

iii. *Low water content lenses:* Low water (below 45%) thin lenses as bandage lenses in disorders of lids such as trichiasis causing trauma to cornea.

Silicone Hydrogels

Silicon hydrogels are new generation lenses with significantly lower level of hypoxia related effects compared to the leading EW hydrogel lenses. They also have lower level of bacterial binding with them.

Collagen Shields

Their main function is drug delivery. Shields soaked in the drug, mostly antibiotics are applied to the eye in case like bacterial ulcers, post PK, etc. where the drug is released in high concentration.

High Dk RGP

All corneal abnormalities leading to irregular astigmatism or high amounts of astigmatism will benefit visually only with rigid lenses. Conditions like postkeratitis cornea, post PK, traumatic cornea or keratoconus, the cornea is already compromised so lenses with maximum Dk should be fitted to these patients to prevent further insult to the cornea (Fig. 17.2).

Selection of the Lens

The lens type is selected on the following criterias:

Oxygen Transmissibility

High water content, thin mid water content lenses, silicone hydrogels or high Dk RGP lenses give the best transmissibility. Lenses which have to be worn for extended periods should be selected from either of these materials.

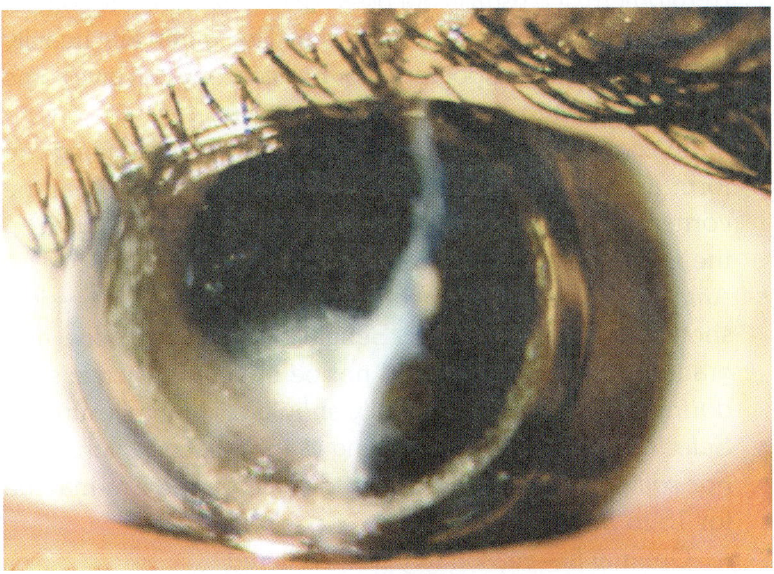

Fig. 17.2: Perforated cornea with RGP

Select high water contact lens in eye conditions where the lens has to act as a splint. RGP lenses as discussed earlier are for irregular compromised corneas to achieve better vision .

Diameter

Soft bandage lenses are usually larger in diameter usually 14.0 to 15.0 mm.

Power

Bandage lenses are usually plano in power (Fig. 17.1).

Disposable Lenses or FRP Lenses

Disposable lenses or FRP lenses are selected as bandage lenses. Therapeutic lenses should be preferably discarded after every use. They are nowadays rarely cleaned and reinserted. Deposits formation is very likely and heavy in such eye conditions.

Fitting Guidelines

- *Keratometry* it is usually not possible to determine the corneal curvature in such eye conditions. The mires are heavily distorted. Corneal topography or Keratoscopy can give some useful information in selecting curvatures.

  In case of traumatic corneas, the good eye K reading can form a base line to start with, on the assumption that the corneal curvature may have been same before trauma in the eye to be fitted with contact lens.
- *Anterior segment assessment* is important. Staining if possible should be done with rose Bengal dye and recorded and graded. Also the eye should not be in acute infective state during fitting. Tear film stability should also be measured.
- *Select the type of lens* according to the eye condition
- *For soft lenses*—allow the lens to settle on the eye may be for 15 to 20 minutes
  - Optimal fit—reasonably well centered
  - Complete coverage of the cornea

- Movement slightly restricted at the same time does not allow the debris to accumulate behind. About 0.3 to 0.5 mm with each blink.
- Observe the eye condition after 4 hours, then 24 hours of wear. Ensure there is no complication developing because of the lens and the wound has started healing.
- In most cases the bandage lens is worn for short periods of extended wear, *regular follow-ups are important.*
- It is the practitioner who inserts and removes these lenses whenever needed. However, the patient should also be explained the emergency removal technique and contact lens care and maintenance. He should have a container with the soaking solution at hand with him.

- *RGP* – Measure the good eyes keratometry in case of uniocular disorders as base line.
  - The fitting is done on hit and trial basis.
  - There should not be excessive bearing or clearing areas. The tears should exchange properly and debris should also not collect behind the lens
  - Achieve a stable centered lens.

Some of the pathologies and the approximate length of the time the therapeutic lenses are used.

Bullous keratopathy	Pain relief from rupture of bullae	HWC soft lens FRP lenses Silicone hydrogels	> 12 months
Recurrent erosion	Splints epithelium Relieves pain	HWC soft lens Silicone hydrogels	2 to 3 months
Filamentary keratitis	Foreign body sensation relief from filaments	HWC, MWC soft lenses	2 weeks
Corneal perforation	To seal the leak	MWC soft lens	Usually maximum upto 1 month

Contd...

Contd...

Entropion / trichaisis	Protection of cornea from aberration	Thin MWC soft lens FRP	Till surgical intervention
Postkeratoplasty	As splint	HWC soft lenses Silicone hydrogels	Till heals 1 week to 1 month

COLORED CONTACT LENSES (Fig. 17.3)

Colored soft lenses are also used in practice. Besides cosmetic reasons, they also form a part of therapeutic lenses.
Reasons to fit a soft colored lenses contact lens are:

- Cosmetic reasons
- Traumatic and post surgical scars
- Pthisis bulbi
- Aniridia
- Albinism
- Diplopia
- Amblyopia therapy.

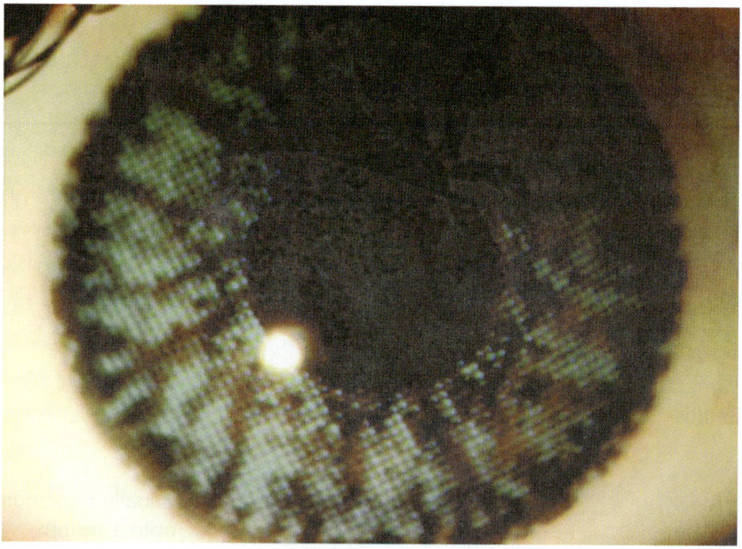

Fig. 17.3: Colored contact lens

The tints used in practice are of three types:

1. Visibility tint
2. Cosmetic tints
3. Prosthetic tints.

Visibility (Handling) Tint

Soft lenses are usually white and transparent. Certain tints, like the light blue or green transparent tints are added to improve the visibility of the lens to the patient during lens handling procedures.

These do not affect the eye color when worn.

Cosmetic Tint

They are used to enhance or change the eye color. They are available in plain or in powers. They are of two types (Figs 17.4A and B):

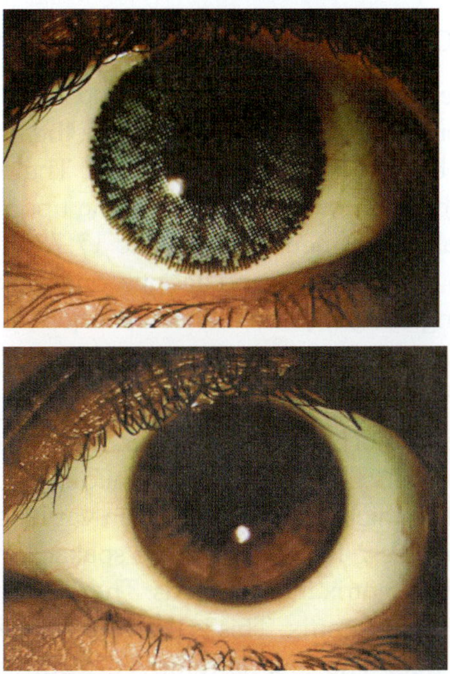

Figs 17.4A and B: (A) Cosmetic lens, (B) without cosmetic lens

- Transparent
- Opaque

The tinted zone of the soft lens covers the iris color and changes or enhances it.

Transparent Tints

These lenses transmit 70% of the light. They are available in various shades. The tint is in the form of a concentric ring, which has a clear centre pupil.

Opaque Tint

They absorb or reflect all incoming light, therefore used to completely change or mask the underlying eye color. They have an iris pattern, with a clear central pupil. The clear pupil is typically 5 mm in diameter.

Prosthetic Contact Lenses

They are fitted to enhance the appearance of a damaged or injured eye or as an occluder in amblyopia therapy.

They can be clear center or dark center. The pupillary zone selected can be clear or opaque depending upon the cosmetic and the visual requirement (Figs 17.5 to 17.7).

Even with best materials and designs, one cannot match the normal looking eye yet can enhance their quality of life.

Tinting Methods

- *Dye dispersion:* The dye is added to the monomer, before polymerization. The final color is uniform and throughout the lens. The thickness of the lens can vary the shade.
- *Vat dye process:* The lens is firstly soaked in a hypotonic solution. The matrix thus expands. The water-soluble dye is absorbed in the matrix. This is then converted into a water insoluble dye. The lens is removed from the hypotonic solution. The matrix shrinks and the dye is trapped.

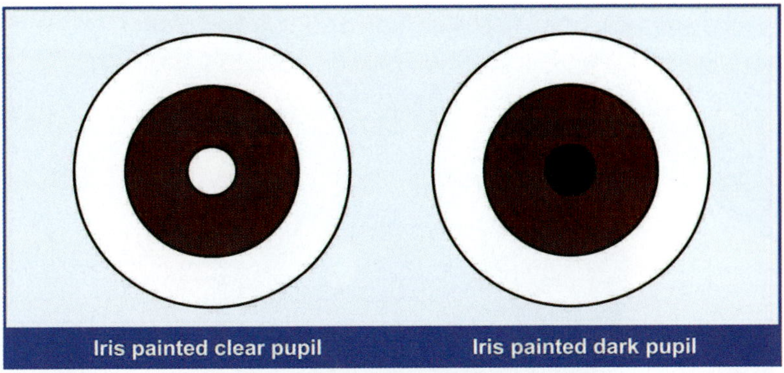

Fig. 17.5: Prosthetic lens: Iris painted clear pupil and iris painted opaque pupil

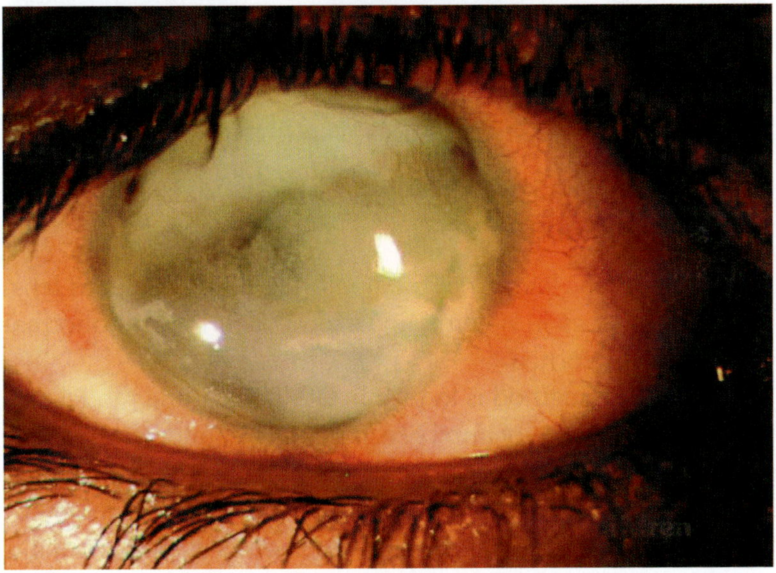

Fig. 17.6: Opaque and unsightly cornea

- *Covalent bonding:* The lens surface is reacted with the dye and then bonded chemically to the matrix.
- *Print transfer process:* The tint or the pattern is printed onto the surface of the lens.

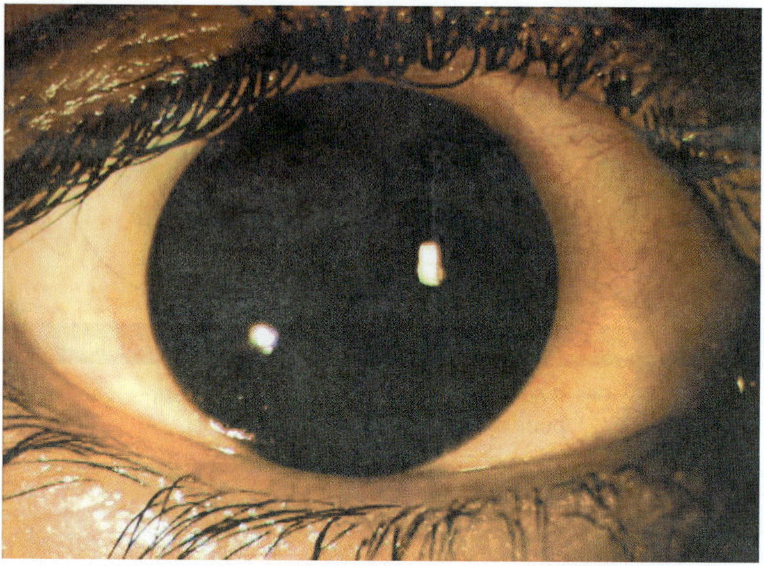

Fig. 17.7: Dark pupil iris painted lens covering the opacity

Fitting Guidelines for Prosthetic Lens (Figs 17.8A and B)

Fitting prosthetic lens is not different from fitting standard lens. The difficulty lies in determining a proper fit for an abnormal iris, pupil and cornea.

The easiest method is to take healthy eye as the model and take measurements of pupil size, iris diameter and keratometry. Evaluate the condition and the health of the eye. Finally match the colors—select from the available colors closest to the eye.

Several times there are limited parameters available but it is usually sufficient for most of the eyes. One may have to order a custom design lens parameters and eye shade for an individual with matching pupil and iris size.

Lens Care

Lens care systems are same for colored lenses. One must check manufacturer's recommendations like some lenses are not compatible with peroxide systems.

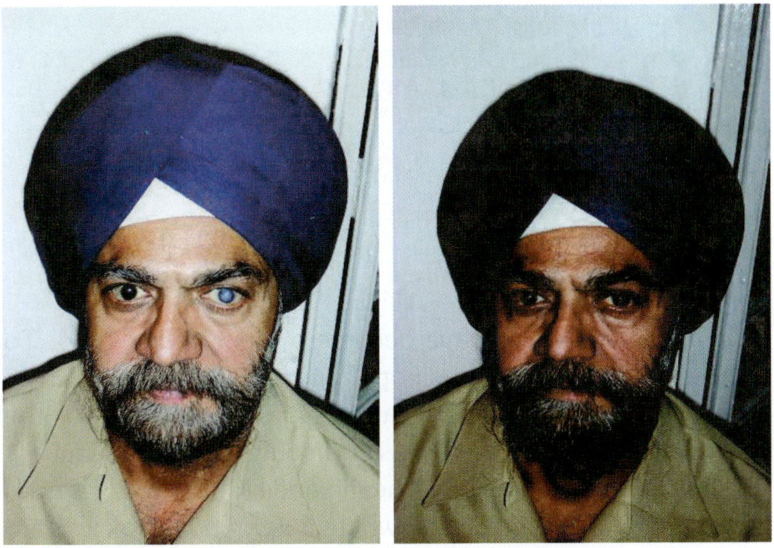

Figs 17.8A and B: (A) Opaque cornea, and (B) Cosmetic CL on opaque cornea

Patient should be explained all do's and don'ts like any lens wearer would be. It is common to see usage and exchange of different colors between friends and family members. One should be warned against this. If the colored lens wear has to be for occasions then one should be explained the daily replacement of soaking solution, even if the lens is not worn that day.

Disposables are Gaining Popularity

It is usually seen that patients who wear different colored lenses are less attentive to their cleaning regimen. They may have an extra colored lens pair for occasions. It is safer to recommend disposable lenses to these patients.

18 Extended Wear Lenses

Extended wear lenses have become a reality since 1984. To some extent, the growth and popularity of extended wear lenses had reduced after some years of launch because of the unfortunate experiences of risks and complication incidences.

Understanding the corneal health and requirement, reduced the popularity. It is time again where we can now look forward to safe extended wear with newer materials and technologies.

The patient's desire is always to sleep in lenses. The reduced requirements in terms of lens care, saving time each morning and evening and also the convenience of not having to remove and insert lenses, are major factors. Another often cited reason is the vulnerability of not being able to see during the middle of the night in the event of an emergency, and the nuisance of simply not being able to read a clock. Less lens care also means reduced expenditure on disinfection systems, and thus savings for the patient.

The practitioner must understand the patient's desire for less hassle—for simplification - and evaluate the risks and the benefits associated with extended wear in order to provide appropriate recommendations to the patient.

But the history of extended wear is far from problem free. Soon after the introduction in the late seventies and early eighties, it became apparent that certain adverse reactions occurred in higher frequency with extended wear. In particular, inflammatory reactions such as acute red eye and giant papillary conjunctivitis were frequent causes of disruption to lens wear.

Loss of sight and pain associated with corneal ulcers also presented a troublesome threat to public health.

The mechanism implicated by scientists to explain these changes is hypoxia.

Let us revise the oxygen requirements in open and closed eye conditions.

Under open eye conditions, oxygen is derived from

- The atmosphere via the tear film.
- The posterior cornea may derive some oxygen from the aqueous.

During eye closure

- The palpebral conjunctiva provides the major component of the corneal oxygen supply,
- Although the limbal blood vessels and the aqueous humor may provide small amounts.

Some changes that occur in closed eye are

a. The available oxygen under closed eye conditions amounts to approximately one-third of that during open eye conditions
b. The temperature of cornea increases by 3 to 4 degrees Celsius. The cornea thus needs more oxygen with higher temperatures.
c. There is diminished tear production during sleep.
d. The pH of the tears shifts to acid at night and the soft lens tightens up in acidic medium.

It can be seen that, during eye closure with wear of a high Dk/t lens, Fatt predicted that the oxygen tension would dip slightly below 40 mm Hg across the cornea. With eye closure and a low Dk/t lens, he predicted that the tension would fall to nearly zero at the posterior epithelium, which could be a serious concern for severe hypoxic consequences.

When the eye is closed the picture becomes a little more complex. First, there is approximately 4% swelling in the absence of a contact lens, meaning that the baseline is no longer zero swelling. Holden and Mertz found that the critical Dk/t to give 4% swelling and no more during overnight wear is 87 +/ –3 barrer/cm. An alternative criterion suggested by Holden and Mertz was to use the day 2 residual swelling. This is the relative edema after the eye has been opened during the day following overnight wear. The cornea will normally recover from upto 8% of edema under open eye conditions. A critical value of Dk/t to of 34 was established for zero day 2 residual swelling.

Practitioners should consider the question of oxygen performance very carefully in fitting patients, particularly when fitting for extended wear .

It is not only the oxygen flux but also the mechanical properties of the lens, which should also give safe; wear to the eye in closed eye conditions.

Patient Selection

1. Well-motivated patients
2. Good compliance
3. Any medical condition that makes putting and taking off lenses difficult.
4. Any anomaly that needs the lenses to be worn continuously
5. In infants and toddlers where insertion and removal by parents is difficult whenever the child takes a nap.
6. As therapeutic/bandage lenses.
7. Occupational need.

Rejection of Patients for Extended Wear

1. Dry eyes
2. Any ocular infection or lid abnormality
3. Previous history of infections or compliance problems

Oxygen performance for a given individual lens wearer can be improved by the following strategies:

a. *Lens thickness can be reduced,* e.g. by going to an ultrathin lens rather than a standard thickness lens
b. *Water content is increased*
c. By *increasing movement,* a marginally improved oxygen performance will result
d. *Decreasing the optic zone* size in higher power lenses reduces the maximum thickness to which a lens must be cut for both plus and minus lenses.

Lenses available as extended wear are:

1. Soft lenses
   - High water content > 70%
   - Ultra thin lenses < 0.05 mm
2. RGP lenses
   - Fluorosilicone polymers—high Dk
   - Silicone—acryalate lenses
3. Silicone hydrogels.

For extended wear, currently available non-silicone materials have been insufficient to meet the cornea's need adequately. Now, we see the possibility of new materials in development having the required properties to meet the cornea's needs. Silicone elastomer lenses of the past produced excellent oxygen performance but were virtually not wearable because of mechanical and surface properties like poor wettability.

Silicone Hydrogel Contact Lenses for Extended Wear or Continuous Wear

Newer lens materials have been developed to improve the oxygen performance. The latest is the silicon hydrogel, which can be worn on continuous basis *from daily wear to 30 days continuously.*

It is a combination of silicone with high oxygen permeability and hydrogel with excellent fluid transport. The unique surfacing property (AerGel technology) transforms the hydrophobic silicone lens into hydrophilic silicate smooth surface with consistent wettability.

Newer technologies now also have silicone hydrogel materials with improved wettability.

The novel properties of silicone hydrogel materials, is elimination of lens-induced hypoxia and its associated effects (e.g. corneal swelling, microcysts, hyperemia and vascularization).

It has increased ability to overcome common contact lens-related problems such as bacterial binding, dehydration and mechanical complications.

Silicone hydrogels have superior water retention as a result of their low water content, but some silicone hydrogels retain water more efficiently than others.

Overall silicone hydrogel lenses *deposit low levels of prote*in compared to non-silicone lenses Corneal swelling, one of the most acute complications of lens-induced hypoxia, occurs to a far less extent during overnight wear with silicone hydrogels compared to conventional hydrogels. Silicone hydrogels can have a positive effect on endothelial cell density in subjects who had previously worn low-Dk lenses and have the potential to relieve some polymegethism and pleomorphism in eyes with a long history of hydrogel.

Silicone-rubber based flexible contact lenses are not new, with silicone-elastomeric lenses being used for therapeutic and pediatric applications for many years. These lenses offer exceptional oxygen transmission and durability, but a number of major limitations are associated with their use in clinical practice. Fluid is unable to flow through these lens materials, resulting in frequent lens binding to the ocular surface and the lens surfaces are extremely hydrophobic, resulting in *marked lipid deposition*.

In silicone-hydrogel materials, silicone rubber is combined with conventional hydrogel monomers. The silicone component of these lens materials provides extremely high oxygen permeability, while the hydrogel component facilitates flexibility, wettability and fluid transport, which aids lens movement. The process of combining conventional hydrogel monomers with silicone proved to be an enormous challenge and it has taken over 20 years of considerable intellectual input and financial resources for these materials and designs to be created. Indeed, the process of combining these monomers has been linked to efforts of combining oil with water, while maintaining optical clarity.

Silicone hydrogel lenses have now removed these obstacles to healthy use of contact lenses for extended wear. *Their high-DK values provide the best oxygenation for the cornea, relieving those common problems*. The new contact lenses also appear to resist protein build up more effectively. The lens surface works to deter bacteria adhesion, which contributes to a decreased chance of microbial infection. While patients who wear mid-water lenses can also enjoy the same advantages of overnight wear, it comes with a much lesser degree of *safety* than overnight wear with silicone hydrogel lenses. High-Dk/t lenses minimizes hypoxic corneal changes that include microcysts, limbal hyperemia and neovascularization

Three silicone hydrogel lens materials are currently commercially available, with their major features being summarized in Table 18.1.

Table 18.1: Silicone hydrogel lens materials

Proprietary name	*Pure vision*	*Focus night and day*	*Acuvue advance*
United States adopted name	Balafilcon A	Lotrafilcon A	Galyfilcon A
Manufacturer	Bausch & Lomb	CIBA Vision	Vistakon
Center thickness (@ -3.00 D) mm	0.09	0.08	0.07
Water content	36%	24%	47%

Contd...

Contd...

Proprietary name	*Pure vision*	*Focus night and day*	*Acuvue advance*
Oxygen permeability ($\times 10^{-11}$)	99	140	60
Oxygen transmissibility ($\times 10^{-9}$)	110	175	86
Modulus	148	238	65
Surface treatment	Plasma oxidation, producing glassy islands	25 nm plasma coating with high refractive index	No surface treatment. Internal wetting agent (PVP)
FDA Group	III	I	I
Principal monomers	NVP, TPVC, NCVE, PBVC	DMA, TRIS, siloxane macromer	Unpublished

DMA *N,N*-dimethylacrylamide; HEMA 2-hydroxyethylmethacrylate; MA methacrylic acid; NVP N-vinyl pyrrolidone; TPVC tris-(trimethylsiloxysilyl) propylvinyl carbamate; NCVE *N*-carboxyvinyl ester; PBVC poly [dimethylsiloxyl] di [silylbutanol] bis[vinyl carbamate]; PVP polyvinyl pyrrolidone

In silicone hydrogels, *the relationship between Dk and water content* is the opposite. Here higher water content implies lower Dk. With these lenses Dk increases significantly as the silicone content—not water content—of the lens increases. The Dk values of silicone hydrogel contact lenses are much higher than those of older soft lens materials.

Silicone, by nature, is *intensely hydrophobia*. A lens made with pure silicone would have tremendous oxygen transmission, but would be unwearable. The lens wouldn't wet at all. To make the surfaces of silicone hydrogel lens materials hydrophilic, techniques incorporating plasma into the surface processing of the lens have been developed. These surface treatments mask the hydrophobic silicone from the tear film, increasing the surface wettability of the materials and reducing lipid deposition.

Despite the advances in care systems, mid-water contact lenses are much more prone to deposits than are silicone hydrogels. Combined with frequent replacement schedules and proper care systems, wearers of silicone hydrogels are *relatively immune to protein deposition*.

Silicone hydrogels offer benefits that conventional lenses don't. Continuous wear contact lenses can prove especially useful for *certain vocations or professions*. Members of the emergency work force (medical personnel, fire fighters and the police) often work unpredictable hours and schedules. They may benefit from immediate clear vision on waking. Other shift workers may appreciate similar advantages. Additionally, increasing numbers of patients enjoy active outdoor life-styles, where patients are unable to disinfect or handle their contact lenses in a hygienic manner.

Symptoms of *discomfort and dryness* often reported by mid-water lens wearers are significantly reduced for silicone hydrogels.

Meanwhile, the contact lens industry is correcting some of the early surprises associated with silicone hydrogels such as solution incompatibility. Furthermore, silicone hydrogels should reduce modulus-related surprises such as mucin-balls, superior epithelial arcuate lesions (SEALs), contact lens papillary conjunctivitis (CLPC) and conjunctival epithelial flaps.

Finally, the contact lens market is experiencing a notable shift in silicone hydrogel prescribing away from continuous wear toward daily wear. This shift toward daily wear should further enhance clinical safety for patients wearing silicone hydrogel lenses.

In all probability, every major contact lens manufacturer will release silicone-based hydrogels over the next 10 years. These materials will address the concerns seen in the current offerings of lenses.

Little doubt exists that silicone hydrogel materials will displace conventional contact lens materials over time for both daily and overnight wear. Silicone hydrogel lenses have improved physiological performance, excellent handling characteristics and improved comfort, making them as close to the ideal contact lens material as we have today.

Silicone Hydrogel Benefits at a Glance

- FDA-approved continuous wear for upto 30 days
- Minimal corneal complications due to lens material
- Highest oxygen transmission, which is best for cornea health
- Comfortable
- Convenient
- Makes a good bandage lens.

19 Lens Dispensing

After the lens is made for the patient the practitioner should follow the following routine when the patient visits the clinic to pick up his lens.

While dispensing the practitioner should verify the parameters of the lens on the eye and recheck the on eye fitting and vision because it is the responsibility of the practitioner to ensure that the lenses are correct and in good condition.

The following should be assessed to confirm the performance of the lens on the eye.

1. Vision
2. Comfort
3. Fitting

Vision Assessment

- Record visual acuity with lenses uniocularly and binocularly
- Do over refraction
- During over refraction check for any deficiencies or any residual astigmatism.

Fitting Assessment

- Check fitting, movement, centering, and coverage for soft lenses
- Check static and dynamic fitting for RGP lenses.

Lens Quality

- Assure that the parameters are correct
- The surface has proper wettability
- There is no lens chip/tear
- The edges of the RGP lens are smooth and rounded off.

Ocular Condition

- Ensure that there is no corneal insult
- That there are no toxicity reactions with the solutions to be advised.

Modification/Replacement

- If the lens is found to be having any power or fitting error the lens should be reordered
- If there is marginal error in fitting and power the lens can be dispensed provided it is not going to cause any physiological damage to the cornea
- RGP lenses can be modified like adding little minus power, reducing diameter, flattening peripheral curves to make adjustments in fitting errors on the dispensing visit.

This is also the time when the patient should be given instructions on insertion/removal and care of the lenses. Patient should also be explained adaptive symptoms. The detail of instructions is dealt in the next chapter.

20 Contact Lens Care Systems

When the lens is received from the manufacturer it is sterile, so where does the infection come from. Clearly, most of the complications with contact lens are because of the poor compliance and improper usage of the lens care systems. It is the responsibility of the practitioner to understand first and then explain the proper usage of each care system.

Care systems or solutions used for contact lenses are ample in the market today. The purpose of this chapter is to understand the function of each constituent.

The Purpose and Objective of a Lens Care System

- To maintain comfort
- Provide good vision
- Maintain eye health
- Maintain lens hydration and parameters stability

With every wear the lens attracts proteins, lipids, mucins, minerals from the eye, and cosmetics, microorganisms and contaminants from external sources like hands.

These accumulate on the lens and form a coating called the biofilm. The lens undergoes changes in parameters due to this, leading to complications like decreased comfort, decreased vision, reduced wearing time, inflammation and infections.

The purpose of the lens care is thus to make the lens wear safe for the eye.

A Typical Lens Care System

Cleaning

It removes microorganisms and loose debris and prepares lens for disinfection.

Rinsing

Removes the cleaner and debris after cleaning.

Disinfection

Kills microorganisms, which may remain on the lens.

Enzymatic Cleaning

Removes firmly attached proteins from lens surface.

Lubricating

Rewet the lens surface while the lens is being worn.

Chemical Properties of Care Products

All lens care systems should:
- Adequately perform cleaning, rinsing and disinfection
- Be nontoxic and harmless to ocular tissues
- Be compatible with lenses and cause no changes in parameters
- Be simple to use
- Be affordable.

THE LENS CARE SOLUTIONS HAVE FOLLOWING PROPERTIES AND INGREDIENTS

Tonicity—0.9% NaCl

The standard of tonicity is 0.9% NaCl (sodium chloride). Solutions are formulated to be isotonic in order to maintain the water balance of the contact lenses and the ocular tissues.

Sodium chloride—NaCl is the primary tonicity agent used in lens care formulations.

Degree of Acidity/Basicity pH—6.6 to 7.8 Comfort Range

The average pH of human tears is from 7.0 to 7.4. Solutions that are outside the eye's comfort range of 6.6 to 7.8 will cause discomfort, usually burning and stinging when put in the eye.

Small quantities of HCl (hydrochloric acid) and NaOH (sodium hydroxide) are common ingredients needed to adjust the pH.

Buffering Agent—Maintain pH

Atmospheric carbon dioxide can enter into the open bottles and dissolve in the solution to make carbonic acid. This lowers the pH. Buffers are thus added in the solutions to maintain the pH to comfort levels of 7.0 to 7.4, e.g. borate, phosphate or citrate.

Viscosity—Increase Contact

Viscosity agents are added to the solutions for greater contact with surface, e.g. polyvinyl alcohol, methyl cellulose, hydroxyethyl cellulose, sodium hyaluranate.

Antimicrobial Activity

Solutions have a preservative and a disinfectant.

Preservatives: Resist or prevent microbial growth in solution once opened.

Disinfectants: Control growth of microorganisms in lens care solutions and eliminate harmful organisms from the contact lens.

Safety vs Efficacy of Preservatives and Disinfectants

All solutions must be strong enough to kill microorganisms but at the same time mild enough to harm ocular tissue.

Commonly used Antimicrobial Agents in Contact Lens Solutions

1. *Biguanides:* For example, polyaminopropyl biguanide, polyhexidine. They are chemically similar to chlorhexidine and have large molecules, which are not absorbed by lens material. They are effective against bacteria but not so much against fungi. They are used in low concentrations (0.00005 to 0.0001%).
2. *Polyquad*: Concentration 0.001 - 0.005%. They are also large molecule, which are not absorbed by lens. They are less irritating to the eye and can be used both as preservative and disinfectant.
3. *Hydrogen peroxide:* It is cidal in low conc. 50 -60 ppm. High concentrations of 3% very effective but need to be neutralized before insertion of the lens into the eye.
4. *Sorbic acid:* It is a moderately effective preservative. It has good action at low pH also. It may react with proteins on the lens and cause discoloration.
5. *Benzalkonium chloride:* It has detergent action and causes disruption of cell membrane. It is used in certain eye drops and RGP solutions. It binds to SOFT lens, and cause severe toxic reactions. So no BAK preservative solutions should be used with soft lenses.
6. *Chlorhexidine:* It has cidal action and can cause toxic reactions. It is both used as preservative and disinfectant. It is very effective against fungi, especially when combined with thiomersal.
7. *EDTA:* It is a chelating agent that is it binds with metal ions needed for growth. It has no cidal activity of own.
8. *Quaternary ammonium:* Same action as BAK but has larger molecules so less toxic.
9. *Thiomersal:* It is mercury based, and has cidal action against bacteria and fungi. It is common to see hypersensitivity reactions with thiomersal. It is used in 0.001% as preservative 0.005% as disinfectant.

Surfactants

It is used in cleaners. They bind with loose debris, deposits and microorganisms and form micelles - which are removed easily with rinsing, e.g. poloxamer, isopropyl alcohol, tyloxapol, sodium laurel sulphate.

Stabilizers

They prevent dissociation or degradation of chemical formulation, e.g. phophonic acid, sodium nitrate, sodium stannate.

LENS CARE REGIME STEPS

Cleaning (Figs 20.1 to 20.3)

This process should be done daily. Proper cleaning removes 90% of organisms, so the time the lens reaches the disinfection step there is a significant reduction in microbial contamination.

Cleaners mostly contain—surfactant, viscosity agent, chelating agent, buffer and preservative.

There are some specialty cleaning agents like polymeric beads which have abrasive cleaning agent or isopropyl alcohol for dissolving lipids.

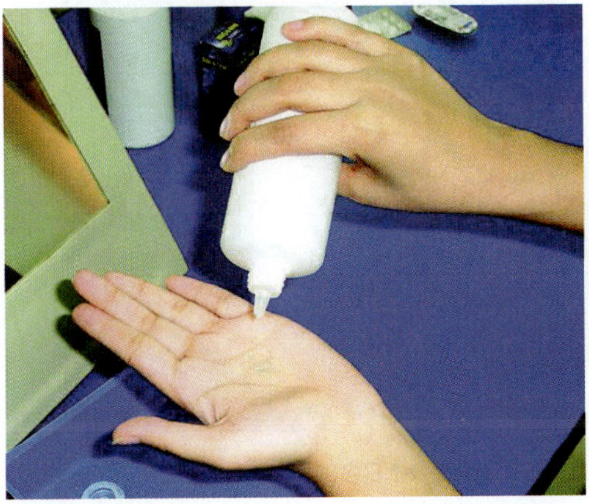

Fig. 20.1: Cleaning solutions

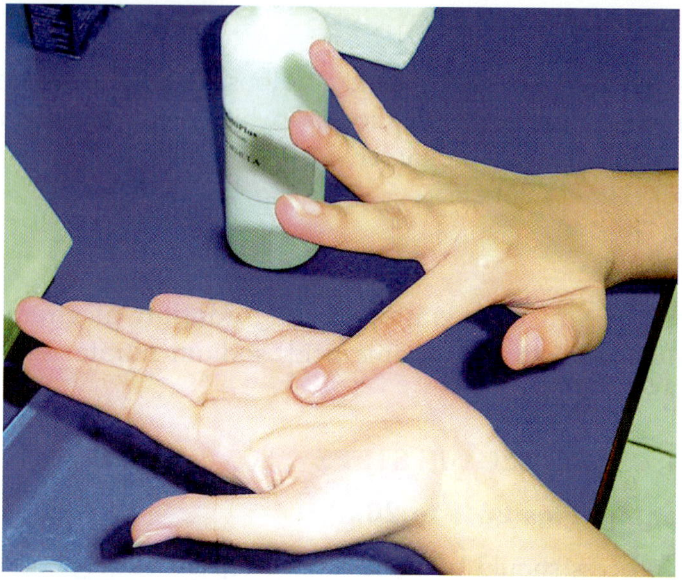

Fig. 20.2: Cleaning of soft lens

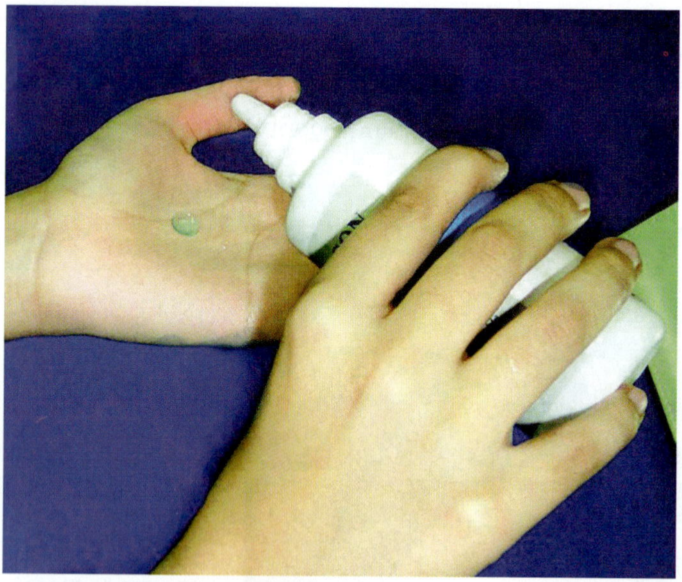

Fig. 20.3: Cleaning of RGP lens

Enzymatic Cleaners (Fig. 20.4)

They also form a part of cleaners by breaking down of proteins. This step is done mostly weekly but depends on the condition of the eye and the deposition. Frequent replacement program lenses may not need this step. It is important to thoroughly rinse the traces of enzyme cleaners from the lenses else they may cause burning and stinging. The lenses tonicity and pH also may have to be re-equilibrated after this step.

Enzymatic cleaners are available in tablet form and contain either of the following compounds:

1. *Papain*—it is an enzyme derived from papaya, may cause ocular irritation, has an unpleasant sulphur odor, is incompatible with some hydrogen peroxide systems and is not so popular
2. *Pancreatin*—is derived from pig pancreas and is effective against protein, lipid and mucin deposit.
3. *Subtilisin*—from bacterial fermentation of bacillus lichniformis. It is compatible with all chemical, thermal and peroxide system of disinfection.

Protein removal has following advantages:

- Regular removal of adherent protein film and deposits
- Increase lens life
- Maintain comfort and vision
- Reduce ocular complications

Emphasis should still be on regular replacement of hydrogels.

Procedure

Clean the lens, prior to enzyme treatment. Soak one tablet of enzyme in 5 ml of soaking solution. Soak the lens in this enzyme solution from 15 mins to 4 hrs (follow manufacturer guidelines). Remove lens and clean very well again. Re-soaking, in fresh solution, may be needed in some type of tablets. The enzyme

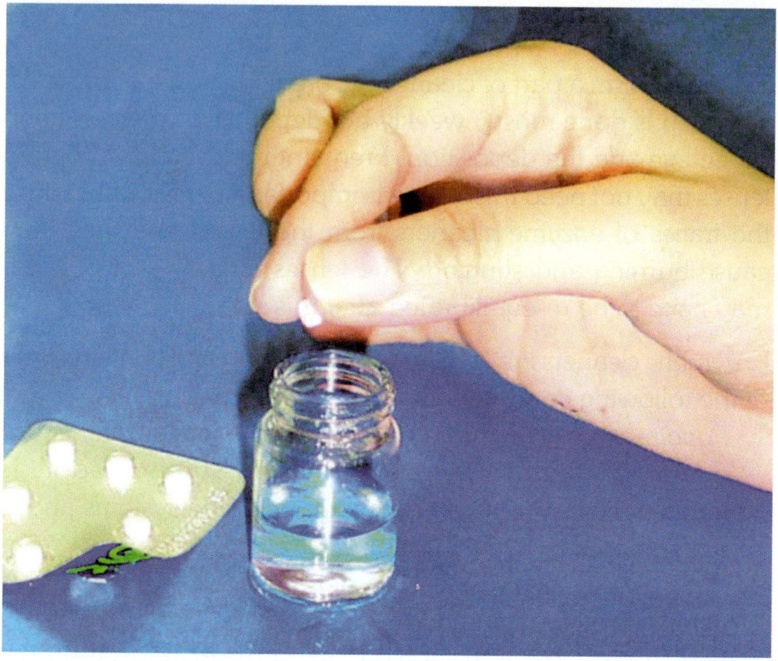

Fig. 20.4: Enzyme treatment

solution is very irritating to the eye and special care should be taken to clean the lens very well before insertion.

RINSING AGENTS (Fig. 20.5)

Saline solutions are the rinsing agents in contact lens care solutions. Their purpose is to rinse to remove cleaner and loose debris. Saline is usually preserved with preservatives so that it does not get contaminated after opening. Unpreserved saline are also used in patients who are sensitive to preservatives. In this case single dose disposable saline units should be used. Unpreserved unit doses are used to avoid toxic reactions.

It has been seen that home made saline can also be prepared. It should be discouraged as home made saline is a great risk and increase the incidence of infections by many folds.

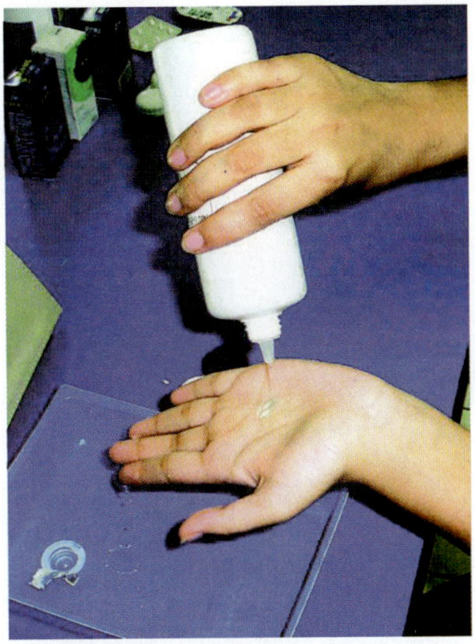

Fig. 20.5: Rinsing solution

DISINFECTION

Disinfection is done after each wear. It protects the eye from infection. With every wear the lens gets contaminated and the common sources of contamination are from hands, cosmetics, tap water, soiled cases.

There are two main methods of disinfection
- Heat
- Chemical

Heat or Thermal Disinfection (Fig. 20.6)

It requires a temperature of 80 degrees for 10 min, followed by cooling period.
Heat disinfection has:

Advantages

Effective against bacteria, fungi, virus and amoeba
- Short disinfection time
- Can be preservative free

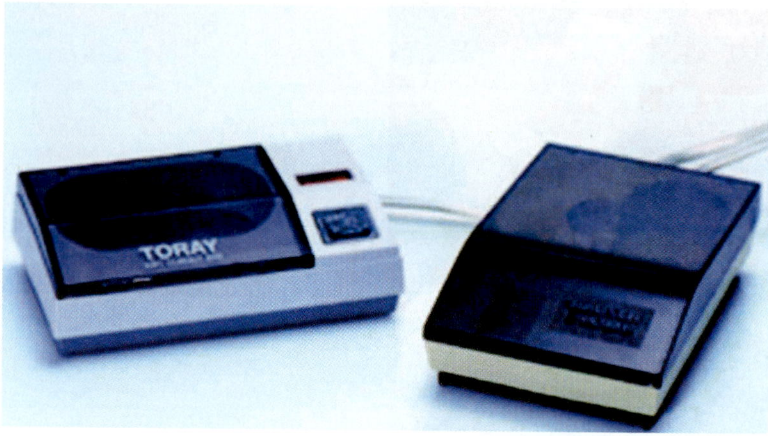

Fig. 20.6: Heating unit/Thermal disinfection

Disadvantages

- Decrease lens life
- Degrades polymer
- Not suited for > 45% water content

Due to its disadvantages the thermal disinfection method is not encouraged these days.

Chemical Sterilization (Figs 20.7A and B)

This method utilizes the property of preservatives and disinfectants to sterilize the lens. Soaking the lens in the soaking

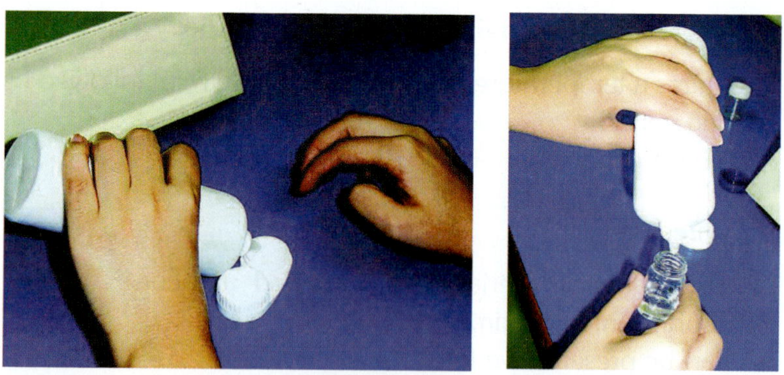

Figs 20.7A and B: Chemical disinfection with soaking solution

solution for an appropriate time sterilizes the lenses. The efficacy depends on preservative type, concentration and the soaking time. Soaking solutions should be discarded after every use. They lose their potency with reuse.

Advantages

- Convenient
- Inexpensive
- Is compatible with most of the modern lens materials
- Most popular method recommended.

Disadvantages

- Preservatives can bind to lens materials and deposits
- Can irritate the cornea
- Patients can develop toxicity reactions
- Certain disinfectants have limited antimicrobial activity.

Oxidative Chemical Disinfection—Hydrogen Peroxide (Fig. 20.8)

Hydrogen peroxide is a very effective disinfectant for a wide range of bacteria and viruses for a relatively short exposure of time (10 minutes approx).

An oxidative reaction occurs whereby the hydrogen peroxide molecule breaks down into free radical, which disrupts the cell wall of the microorganisms. This free radical breaks into water and oxygen further.

$$H_2O_2 \rightarrow \underset{\text{(Free radical)}}{HOOH} \rightarrow H_2O + O_2$$

0.005 to 0.006% is effective as preservative and 3% is effective disinfectant. *This peroxide needs to be neutralized before the lens is placed on the eye.*

Hydrogen peroxide disinfection system has following *advantages:*

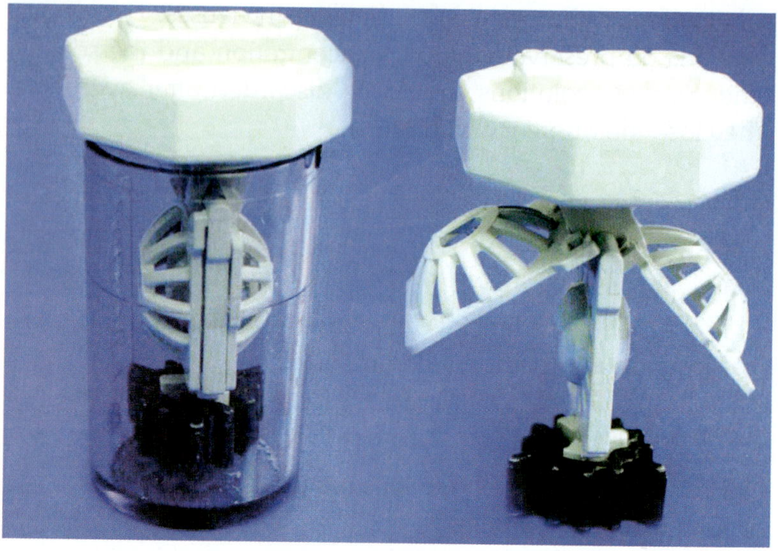

Fig. 20.8: Hydrogen peroxide disinfection system

- It can penetrate deep into pores of lens matrix
- Has very good disinfecting property
- Does not need preservative as has acts as preservative on its own
- It has some cleaning action by breaking down protein and lipid bonds
- It is nontoxic if properly neutralized.

It has following *disadvantages:*

- It may cause ocular toxicity if is not neutralized properly
- It is expensive
- More complex to use
- May effect parameters of FDA group IV lenses.

Neutralization compounds used in peroxide system to convert H_2O_2 into water and oxygen.

1. Catalytic disk of platinum
2. Sodium pyruvate and sodium thiosulphate
3. Catalase.

Based on this the peroxide systems are classified into **one step or two step systems**.

One step peroxide
- is convenient
- pH is close to 6.5
- has inflexible neutralization time
- can be used with protein tabs.

Two step peroxide
- has short neutralization time
- the pH is acidic 3.5
- does have flexible disinfection time.

Lubricating or Rewetting Drops (Fig. 20.9)

Very often contact lens wearing patients complain of dryness. This is usually because of wind, dust, low humidity, heat or even marginal dry eye. Rewetting or lubricating drops need to be added to improve the wettability and prevent the lens from

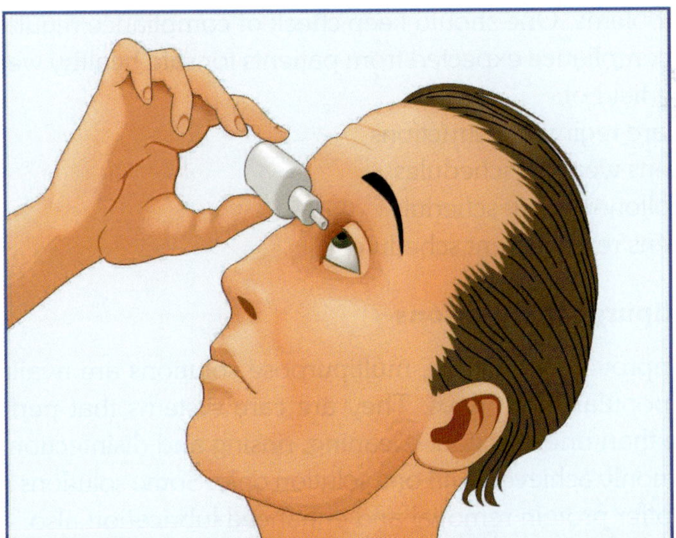

Fig. 20.9: Lubricating /rewetting drops with lens on the eye

drying in the eye. It relieves the symptoms associated with dryness like discomfort reduced wearing time and irritation.

Rewetting drops can be used with the lenses on the eye. Certain artificial eye substitutes or tear supplement drops can also be used, but the preservative in them can bind with the soft lens material and cause problems. So it is safe to use the recommended lubricating drops with the lens on the eye.

Efficacy

The efficacy of disinfection *against bacteria* is—

Heat, 3% H_2O_2, thiomersal 0.002% (4 hrs), dymed 0.005% (4 hrs) polyquad 0.001% (4 hrs).

For fungi and acanthamoeba the effective methods are—Heat, H_2O_2, thiomersal. 002% (4 hrs). Dymed, polyquad, are ineffective against fungi and acanthamoeba.

Compliance

Compliance to maintenance is a very important step to avoid all problems. One should keep check of compliance regularly. The compliance expected from patients for safe healthy wear is in the field of:

1. Care regimen instructions
2. Lens wearing schedules
3. Follow-up visit schedule
4. Lens replacement schedule.

Multipurpose Solutions

To improve compliance, multipurpose solutions are available and popular these days. They are care systems that perform more than one function. Cleaning, rinsing and disinfection are commonly achieved with one solution only. Some solutions may also offer protein removal and enhanced lubrication also.

Disinfection of Trial Lenses

- Disinfect immediately after each use with disinfecting solution.
- Inventory trial lenses should be disinfected at least once a month
- Heat sterilization with preserved saline is also effective, but leads to parameter changes and deposit build up over the period of time.

OVERVIEW OF LENS CARE SYSTEMS

- Cleaning
- Rinsing
- Disinfection

Optional Lens Care Systems

- Enzyme cleaning
- Lubricating.

21 Instructions to Patients

Instruct patient on use of contact lenses during the delivery. A very good fitting may also fail if the patient is not instructed properly on the use and maintenance of the lenses.

Following is the outline of the instructions to be given to each contact lens wearer:

- Insertion and removal
- Cleaning and disinfection procedures
- Wearing schedules
- Normal adaptation symptoms
- Do's and Don'ts of contact lens
- Warning signs
- Follow-up or next appointment

Lens Insertion and Removal Technique

The teaching area should have a table where the instructor sits facing the patient. There should be a mirror, a tray and some lint free tissue papers on this table. The complete range of solution bottles should be at hand. The washbasin should also be at a convenient distance.

Soft Contact Lenses Instructions

The First Basic Step: Wash Hands (Fig. 21.1)

Prior to the teaching session make sure that both the patient and you wash your hand with soap. The soap used should not be cream based. Washing removes all creams and dirt from the hands, which is most likely the source of contamination to the

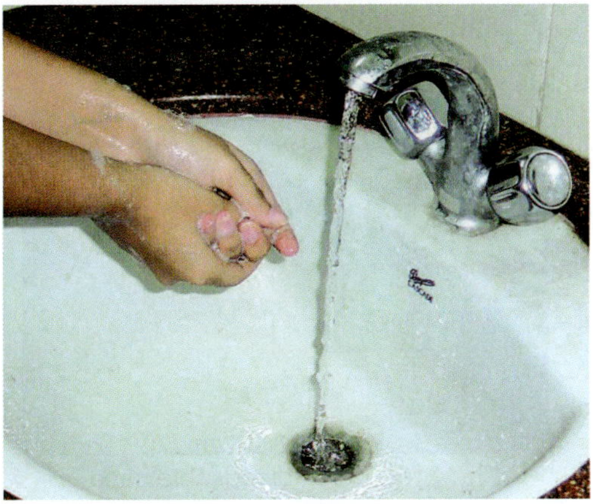

Fig. 21.1: Wash hands

lenses. The hands should then be dried with a lint free towel or tissue papers. Towels with fibers, stick to hands and then get transferred on to lenses.

Remove the Lens from the Container (Figs 21.2 to 21.4)

Rapidly invert the vial and spill the contents into the palm of the other hand. Drain out the solution. Work with one lens at a time, and always begin with the right lens first.

Inside Out

Before applying the lens on the eye, the patient needs to check that the lens is not inside out. To determine this place the lens on the fingertip. Observe the shape of the lens. If the shape is like a bowl that is the edges of the lens are rounded slightly inwards the lens is correct way. If the lens shape is like a saucer that is the edges are rounded slightly outward the lens is inside out.

Certain thick design lenses can also be checked for inside out by TACO test (Fig. 21.5). Hold the lens between the thumb and the index finger. Pinch at the base of the lens gently. Observe

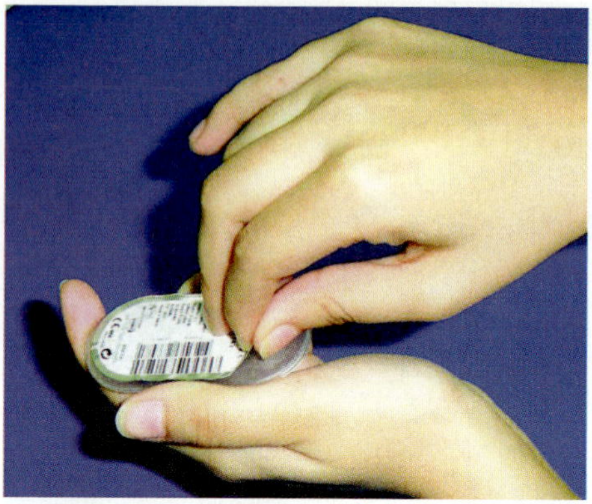

Fig. 21.2: Open disposable case

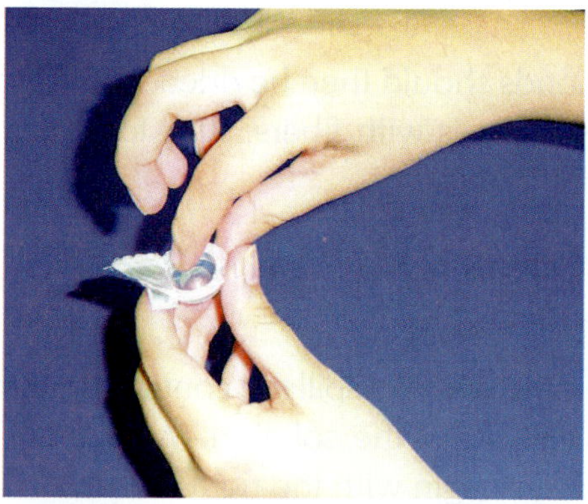

Fig. 21.3: Remove from case

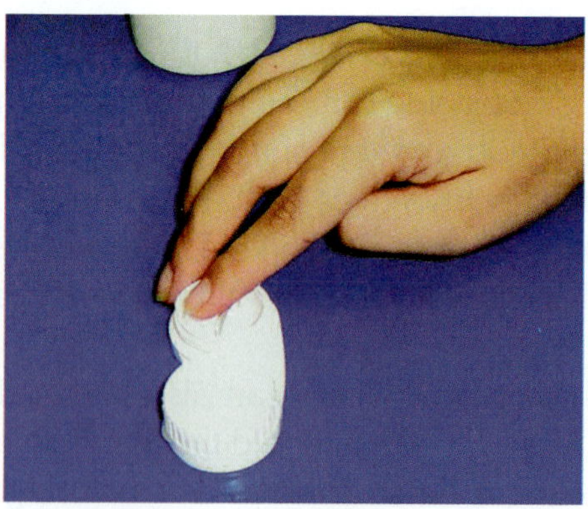

Fig. 21.4: Pick from soaking case

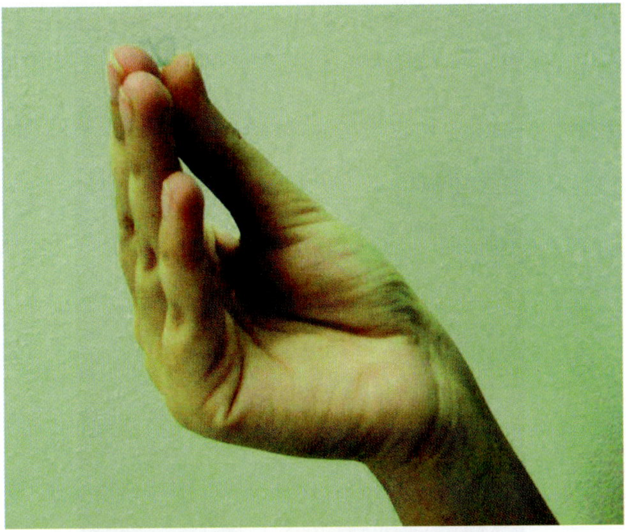

Fig. 21.5: Taco test

the edges. If the edges tend to curl inside the lens is correct way and if the edges tend to curl outside the lens is inside out.

Some manufacturers give a logo or an inside out identification mark at the edge of the lens.

If the lens is inserted incorrect way in the eye it moves more and is usually uncomfortable to the patient.

At this point instruct the patient to instruct for any damage or tear or chip on the lens. This is done by holding the lens on the index finger and observing it all around against the light (Fig. 21.6).

Soft Lens Insertion Technique

Step 1

Patient grasps the upper lid with left hand (non-dominant hand), pulls down the lower lid with middle finger of right hand and holds the lens on the index finger of this hand. (Grasp the upper lid at the lid margin, not above it; else the lids will close by reflex blinking) (Fig. 21.7A).

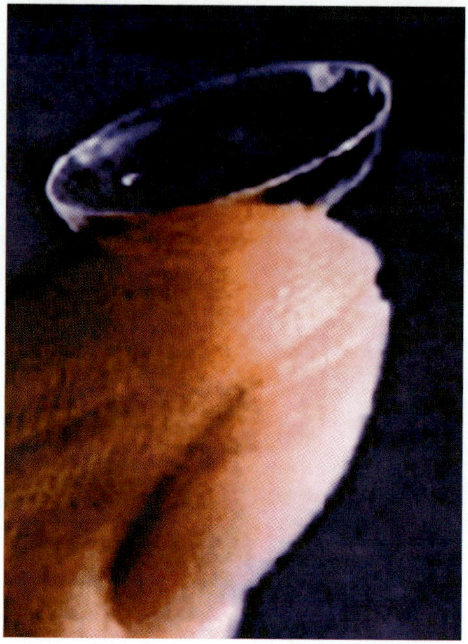

Fig. 21.6: Examine the lens before insertion for any damage or tear

Step 2

The finger holding the lens should be dry. Allow the lens to also air dry slightly before insertion.

Step 3

The patient brings the lens up, looking in the mirror. The lens will self-center with a blink or two, so it has not to be placed directly on to the cornea. More pressure has to be applied to the lens in order to adhere to the eye (Figs 21.7B to D).

Step 4

Once the lens is inserted, have him or her look down before releasing the lids to prevent the lens from being blinked out. Release the lower lid slowly followed by upper lid.

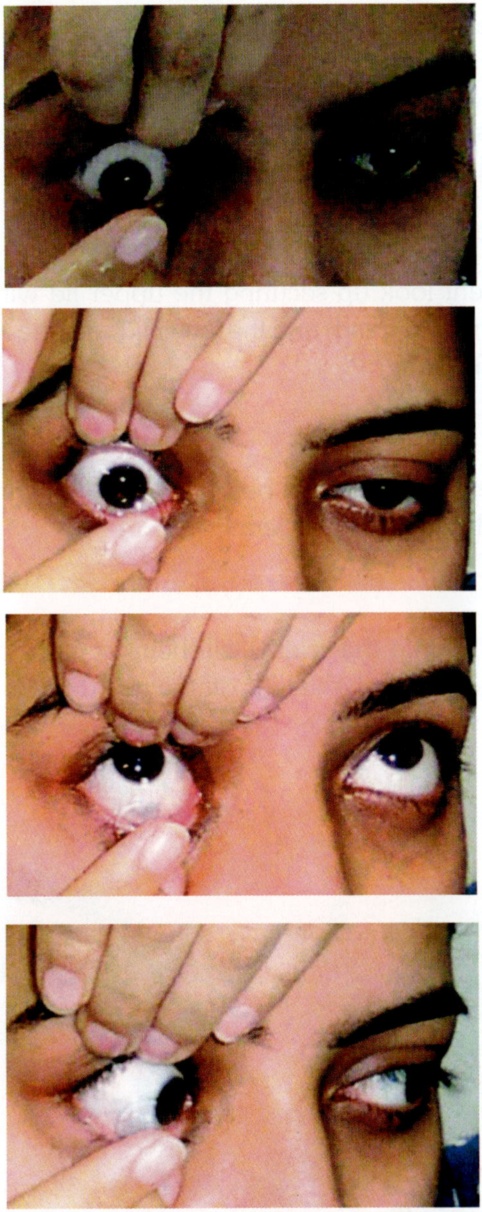

Figs 21.7A to D: Insertion of soft lens: (A) Pull up the upper lid and pull down the lower lid, (B) Place lens directly on the cornea, (C) OR: Place lens looking up, (D) OR: Place lens looking inwards

Soft Lens Removal Technique

Step 1

Check the lens is on place and that it does not feel dry. In case recenter it and instill lubricating drops to rehydrate.

Step 2

Have the patient look up securing the upper lid with the left hand (non-dominant hand) and the lower lid with the right hand or the dominant hand.

Step 3

Using the index finger, of right hand have the patient slide the lens down and out onto the sclera.

Step 4

Once the lens is onto the sclera, tell them to use their thumb and index finger to pinch the lens off the eye (Fig. 21.8).

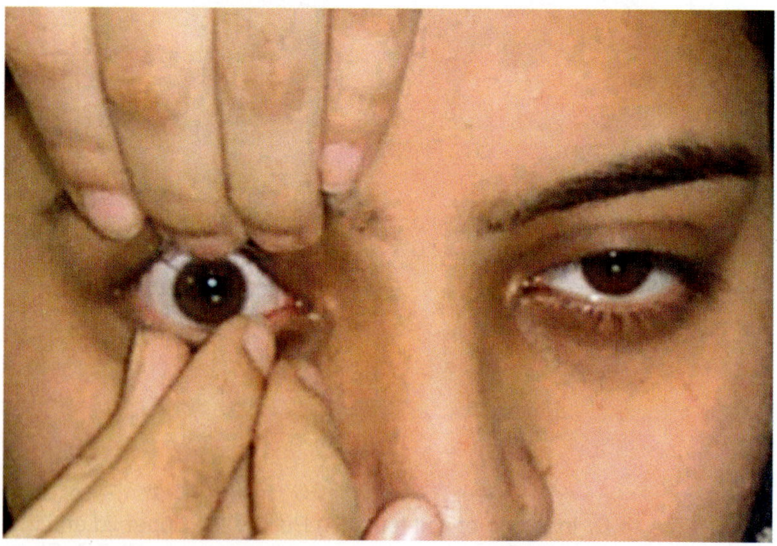

Fig. 21.8: Remove soft: Pinch the lens off with the thumb and the finger

RIGID LENS INSERTION AND REMOVAL

Basic Step—Wash Hands
Insertion Technique

Step 1

Take the left hand over your head and bring it upper eyelid margin and eyelashes holding it securely to the orbital bone. The tight gasp is important.

Step 2

The index finger of the right hand holds the lens and the middle finger pulls down the lower lid.

Step 3

The patient brings the lens up, looking in the upright mirror. Tell the patient to look through the lens and place the lens directly on the cornea.

Step 4

A light touch is needed for the lens to be inserted. The patient should be instructed to keep looking through the lens else the lens will not center on the cornea.

Step 5

Look down release the lower lid first then the upper lid.

Step 6

If displaced teach recentration. Teach the patient to relocate the lens by using two fingers against the lid margin and sliding the lens towards the cornea.

Other method of recentration
Feel the lens with the fingers. With the index and middle finger of the dominant hand hold the lens. Holding the lens, look in

the opposite direction of the lens. Push the lens towards the cornea hold the lens in the center. Don't release the hand. Look straight. The cornea will automatically slide under the lens. Release the hand.

Removal Technique (Fig. 21.9A)

Step 1

Check the lens is in center.

Step 2

Patient has to open his eye wide as possible, have him turn the face so that cornea is slightly nasal in the palpebral opening.

Step 3

Point out the index finger only; roll the other 3 fingers first. Place the index finger of the right hand for right eye, on the outer canthus, elbow pointing straight.

Step 4

Pull up and out, and then forcefully blink. Don't release the force till blink. The lid margins will catch the edge of the lens and the lens will pop out.

Step 5

Remember to put the other hand below to catch the lens.

Using two fingers (Fig. 21.9B)

- With the index fingers of both hands, hold the upper and lower lens edges at the widest points of lens edge.
- Gently push the lower lid upwards, inwards and towards eye, and at the same time push the top lid downwards so that both the lid margins engage lens edges. This enables the lens to slide over the lower lid and out of eye. The lens will now be positioned on the nail of index finger.
- Hold the lens with adjacent finger to prevent it from falling.

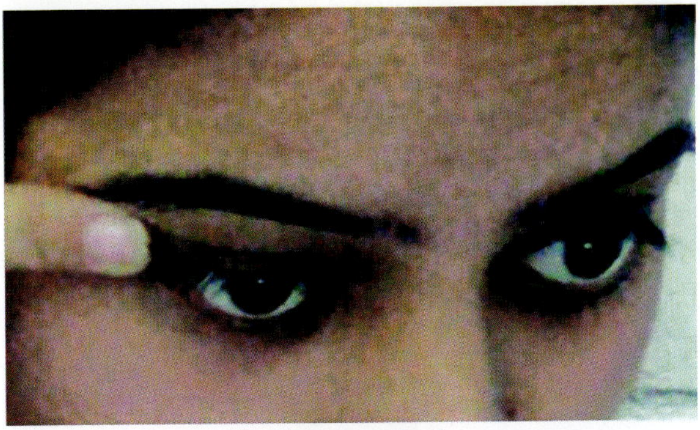

One finger method

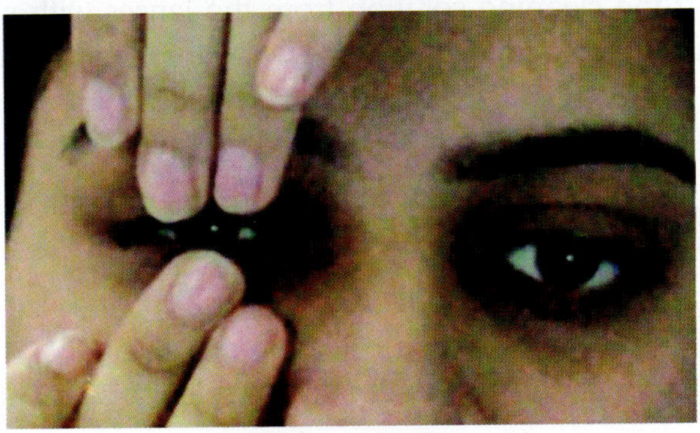

Two finger method

Figs 21.9A and B: Removal of RGP lens

Locating the decentered lens

- Retract the lids, look up, down and right and left to locate the lens.
- Look towards the opposite direction of displaced downwards, if the lens is displaced downwards look upwards look upside and then contact the edge of lens with lid margin.
- Push the lens gently towards the center of the cornea. Keep the other lid retracted and the other eye open during this procedure.
- Do not press but slide the lens edge while pushing the lens.

CLEANING AND DISINFECTION

Soft Contact Lens Care Regimen: Daily Steps

Clean

With the lens on the palm, clean the lens surface by rubbing with two—three drops of surfactant cleaner. Rub in back forth or circular motion for 10 seconds on each side. Clean lenses after, removal at night.

Rinse

Rinse off the cleaning solution from the lenses with saline or multipurpose solutions. Never use water for rinsing soft lenses.

Soaking and Disinfect

Storing the lenses overnight in fresh solution overnight disinfects the lenses.

Rinse

Rinse lenses with saline or multipurpose solution before insertion

Apply the Lens on the Eye

Weekly enzyme treatment. This is optional for disposable lenses.

Rigid Lens Care Regimen: Daily Steps

Clean

With the lens on the palm and with few drops of cleaning solution, rub the lens. Do not do the cleaning within the fingers this can warp or break lenses (Fig. 21.10).

Rinse

Rinse the cleaning solution off the lenses with saline. Some practitioners recommend tap water for rinsing. This is not wrong,

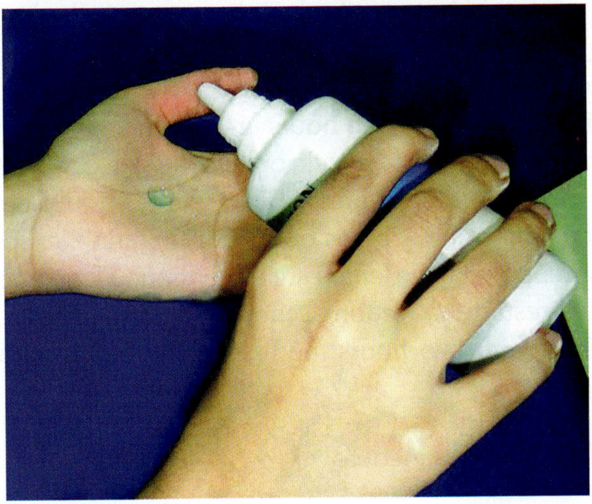

Fig. 21.10: Clean RGP

but contamination from the tap water can be passed on to the eye, especially *Acanthamoeba*.

Soaking and Disinfecting

Storing the lenses overnight (or 4 to 6 hours) disinfects the rigid lenses. Though they can also be dry stored, but then there are chances of contamination and some parameter changes. Dry soaking also leads to poor surface wettability also.

A duplicate pair of lenses can be stored dry and then presoaked and conditioned 4 hours before restarting use.

Rinse

Rinse lenses with saline or tap water before insertion. Use a wetting or conditioning solution before insertion.

Apply on the Eye

Wearing schedules: Follow manufacturers guidelines for recommending wearing schedule to each patient. As a general rule no lens should be worn for long hours or whole day in the beginning. The eye needs 4 to 5 days to adapt to *soft lenses*. It is usual to start with 2 hours the first day increase one or two hours daily till whole waking hours are achieved.

The *rigid lenses* need week or two to get on to regular schedule of whole day wearing. Rigid lenses should be worn daily. They cannot be used as occasional wearing lenses. The sensations reappear if the lenses are discontinued for some days. One should restart the wearing schedule again to readapt. It is usual to start with two hours the first day increasing an hour daily.

Soft Lens Wearning Schedule

Day	*Time*
1st day	2 hours
2nd day	3 hours
3rd day	4 hours
4th day	5 hours
5th day	6 hours
6th day	7 hours
7th day	8 hours

Normal Adaptation Symptoms

It is common for the patient to have mild redness, irritation and discomfort and fluctuating vision when he starts with the lens for the first time. These symptoms are mild with soft lenses and subside in maximum of 5 days.

The symptoms are significant with RGP wearers. It is important to reassure the patient of these normal symptoms, which may be experienced in the initial days.

Some of the symptoms seen normally in beginners using contact lenses are (they usually go away on their own after 7-10 days).

- Tearing

- Lid irritation.
- Difficulty in looking up occasional blurring or disturbance of vision.
- Reduced inclination to extreme eye movements.
- Abnormal head posture
- Excessive blinking
- Photophobia
- Headache
- Lens loss
- Lens displacement

DO'S AND DON'TS OF LENS CARE

Besides the instructions, of care and maintenance and insertion removal the patient should always be added some basic Do's and Don'ts, which will reinforce proper compliance. These also form a part of queries, which usually appear in patients mind during lens wear. *These should be written and discussed with each contact lens wearer to avoid complications.*

Reinforce these Do's

1. Always wash hands, before handling contact lenses.
2. Follow the recommended wearing schedule.
3. Keep the lens case clean and replace as advised.
4. Handle lenses over clean table. Washbasins are risky; lenses can be lost down the drain.
5. Clean and disinfect lenses daily after use.
6. Carry a lens case filled with solution with you while going out of the house.
7. Remove lenses immediately if redness, watering, or irritation start. Consult your practitioner immediately.
8. Wear goggles when moving out in a dusty environment.
9. Follow instructions regarding cosmetics usage with contact lenses.
10. Read all the instructions carefully before starting wear.

Warn these Don'ts

1. Do not sleep with the lenses on the eye, unless recommended.
2. Always replace the soaking solution every night. Don't add over the existing solution.
3. Saline solution if used for rinsing should not be home made.
4. If unpreserved saline is used for rinsing, it should be discarded after every use.
5. Soft lenses cannot tolerate most of the RGP solutions. Read instructions always properly before buying solutions over the counters.
6. Do not change the brands of solutions unless recommended by the practitioner.
7. Buy smaller bottles as far as possible and discard after expiry of opening.
8. Do not touch, the tip of the solution bottle with hands, this might contaminate them (Fig. 21.11).
9. High water content lenses should not be heat disinfected.
10. Some tinted lenses may lose their tint intensity with peroxide systems. Avoid them.
11. Lenses unused for long time should be disinfected always before reuse.
12. Cracked or chipped lens should never be worn.
13. Do not rub your eyes vigorously with lens on the eye.

Reinforce Lens Care Tips

- Always wash and rinse your hands thoroughly before you handle your lenses.
- To avoid getting your lenses mixed up, always apply (or remove) your lenses, one at a time, in the same order.
- Never use eye drops or solutions that are not specifically for contact lenses.
- Do not use saliva to try and wet or clean your lenses.

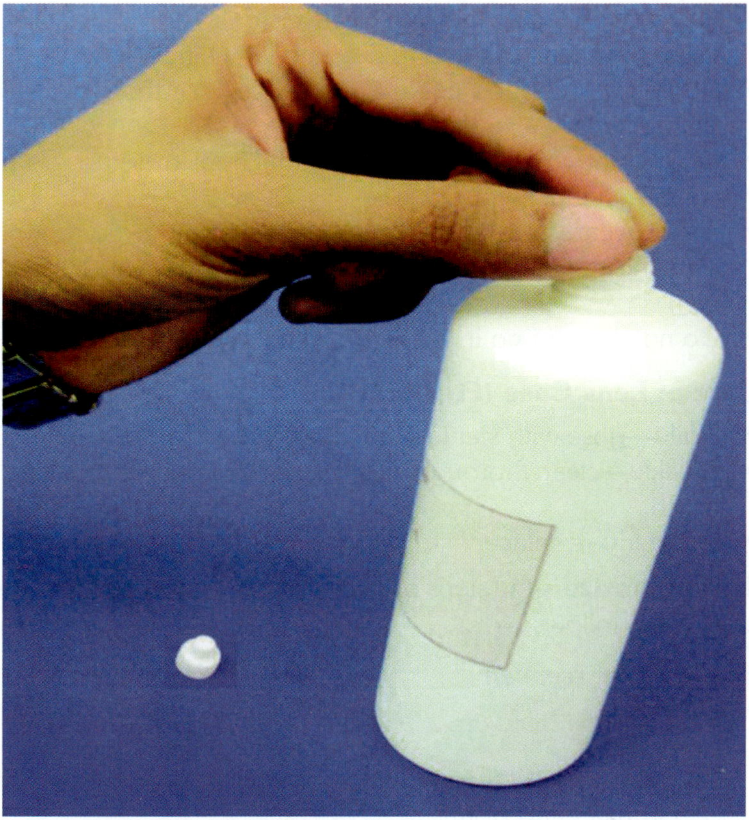

Fig. 21.11: Don't touch the tip of the bottle

- Do not sleep in your lenses (unless you wear lenses that are specifically designed for continuous wear and your eye care professional has prescribed them for that wear schedule).
- Clean, rinse and disinfect your lenses every time you remove them.
- Keep all your solution bottles tightly capped when you're not using them.
- Do not let the tip of solution bottles touch any surface (including your fingers, eyes or lenses).
- Never use expired lens solutions.
- Never re-use lens solutions.

- Never swap lenses with someone else.
- Rinse your lens case every day and let it air dry.
- Replace your lens case every three months (or more frequently).
- Do not let cosmetics like soap, makeup, moisturizers or sunscreen touch your lenses.
- Never wear your lenses when you're going to be around irritating fumes or vapors (paint, hairspray, oven cleaner, etc.)
- Do not swim or go in a hot tub while wearing your lenses.

Care of Lens Case (Fig. 21.12)

- Daily—rinse with sterile saline and allow to air dry
- Weekly—clean thoroughly with surfactant cleaner and tooth brush
- Quarterly—replace.

To summarize—the steps of care systems used in contact lens care are as follows:

Soft lens care regimen

- Daily
  1 clean
  2. Rinse
  3. Disinfect and store
  4. Rinse
  5. Apply to eye
- Weekly
  1. Enzyme

RGP lens regimen

- Daily
  1. Clean
  2. Rinse
  3. Disinfect
  4. Rinse
  5. Apply to eye
- Weekly
  1. Enzymes (optional).

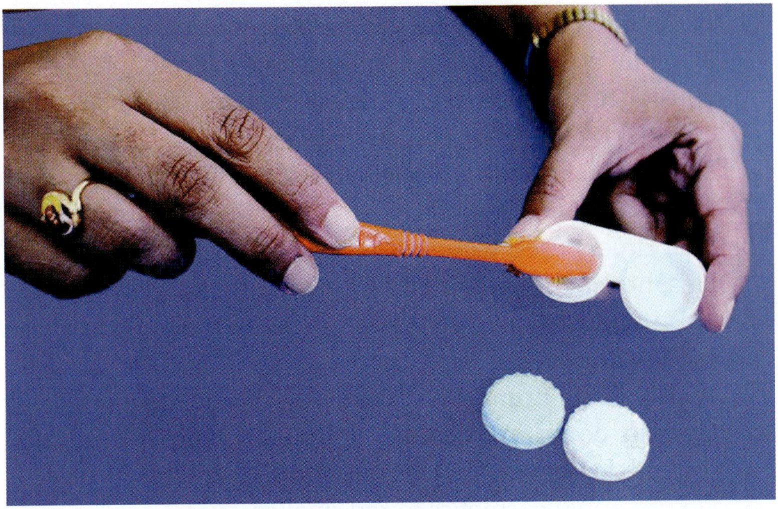

Fig. 21.12: Cleaning of the lens case

USE OF COSMETICS WITH CONTACT LENSES

Almost every body, even males, uses skin care products. Products like hair grooming agents, aftershave lotions, perfumes, deodorants, soaps, creams can have an adverse effect on the contact lens wearer. It may not seem dignified for a contact lens practitioner to discuss the cosmetics with the patient. But it is essential. One must be aware of the cosmetics used by both the sexes and the proper usage along with the lenses should be explained to the wearer. Your carelessness or less information on the cosmetics may cause complications to the wearer.

Hints

1. Cosmetics should be applied after the lenses have been inserted.
2. Cosmetics should be removed after the lenses are removed. Encourage women to use non-greasy, non-creamy lotions to remove and clean the make-up.

3. Patients should never be told to swap, borrow or lens their eye make-up or applicator brushes. Harmful infection causing organisms are transferred this way. If possible change the applicator brush frequently.
4. Lens should not be worn with the sprays and fumes in air. They can cause keratitis.
5. Hair dryers used with soft lenses can cause drying of the lens, hence discomfort and visual hazing
6. False eyelashes can cause blephritis and allergic reaction to the adhesive.
7. Well-known brands of cosmetics should be preferred. Certain companies make hypoallergenic compounds suitable for lenses. They should be chosen.
8. Do not apply cosmetics to red swollen eyes.
9. Apply eyeliner to the outer margins. Use water-soluble brands. Never use *kajal*.
10. Use non-greasy or moisturizer free soaps to wash hands
11. Apply creams and moisturizers to hands after insertion or removal.

Problems—that may Arise from Cosmetics

- Lids—blephritis, allergic response, blocking of ducts
- Cornea—minute abrasions from organic materials and hard particles in the powdered cosmetics
- Tear film—instability due to oily suspensions.

Follow-up or Next Appointment

Fix and reinforce the next appointment on the dispensing visit. Discuss the replacement schedule again before the patient leaves the clinic.

22 Follow Up Care

Contact lenses are medical devices, relatively safe, yet not free from complications. It is known that most of the complications could be prevented if the patient had regular follow up. The drop out rate will also reduce significantly. The patient develops a healthy relation with the practitioner, if he follows up regularly. The follow up date should be emphasized and put in black and white on the day of dispensing.

As a responsible practitioner, one must not neglect the patient after dispensing. Unlike spectacles, the lens is in contact with the eye and the eye can respond negatively. Several times the patient may not be aware of the warning signs and symptoms which may gradually lead to major problems. These can be very comfortably taken care of in the beginning. It is also studied that most of the problems arising due to lenses is because of poor compliance on behalf of the patient. During the follow up visit one can reinforce and rectify that, thus preventing complications and drop outs. Other advantage of follow up is to inform patient about the new technologies and improvement in lens designs and materials. The advancement may be beneficial for the patient, which he would not have ever known if he did not visit you for the follow-up.

THE AFTER CARE ROUTINE

After care, should include both subjective and objective assessment of the lens. Review the information recorded at previous visits. The record file should always be maintained and further information recorded on follow-ups.

Subjective Assessment

Patient Discussion

Start with history—*ask questions*. Be specific and open. Encourage patient to ask questions during the discussion. Recheck the compliance. Before the examination, make a note of the following; these will support you in recommending corrective actions.

- *Lens age:* Every lens has a life. Patients may not be sure of the replacement. Some of the complications may be associated with the aging lens.
- *Wearing habits and time:* Ask- How many hours during the day does one wear lens? How many days during the week? Does one sleep with lenses on?

  If the patient is comfortable wearing lenses during full waking hours, hints that the lens fitting is reasonably good. If the patient admits that he does occasionally sleep with lenses, indicates a thorough examination and need for improved compliance.
- *Review lens care system:* Ask patient to demonstrate. Ask the patient to insert and remove the lens in front of you. Observe his habits and compliance then. Check that he does wash hands; the nails are trimmed and use solutions in proper way and steps.
- *Presence of problems:* Patients may have specific symptoms or at times may neglect some minor complaints are warning signs Ask questions to arrive at conclusions.
  - *Reduced and blurred vision:* Constant or fluctuating, or any specific circumstances when happens
  - *Discomfort:* Foreign body sensation, burning, stinging, dryness, grittiness, itching immediate onset (soon after

insertion) or Delayed onset (after may be an hour of wear), with or without lenses.

- *Environment and occupation:* Air-conditioned office, and computer usage, may lead to dryness.
- *Systemic problems:* Ask if the patient has any systemic problem, which has any correlation with lens wear. Confirm about any intake of drugs and medications.

Objective Assessment

Check up should be done *with lenses on and then after the lenses are removed.* The assessment should be done with the patient attending the clinic with the *lens worn for at least 4 hours before the check up.* This should be explained on the dispensing visit itself. Many of the delayed problems can be identified only after some hours of the wear. If the patient comes for the check up and inserts lenses there it self, some signs may be missed out.

The slit-lamp is the key instrument, which will allow accurate objective assessment.

To start with **check with lenses on:**

Visual Acuity

Record distance and near visual acuity, monocular and binocular. Any deficiency calls for power adjustments. If the patient complains of blurred visual acuity after some hours of wear, rule out corneal edema.

Retinoscopy Over the Lenses

This is the most important technique, after all lens, is a vision-correcting device. The refraction over the lens will guide you if there is any deficiency of power, any over correction, and residual astigmatism. It also hints you about the fitting (clear reflex before and after blink). The reflex through the lens will show deposits and the dirty lens, which calls for replacement. If the optic zone is cutting through the pupil can also be seen now. One can also check if the lenses are switched.

Slit-lamp Examination

Start with examination for surface integrity, deposits, lens surface and edges (chipped). Review the lens fitting. The lens parameters are known to change with the passage of time, especially the soft lenses. These changes can lead to steeper fittings later. Evaluate both static and dynamic fitting with fluorescein dye in case of RGP lenses.

Re-examine without Lenses Next

Slit-lamp Examination

Check the corneal integrity, stain the cornea with the fluorescein dye and look for any aberrations and staining. Make an optical section of the slit and look for any edema. Specular reflection technique should be utilized to note any endothelial changes.

Evert the upper lid now to examine the upper tarsal conjunctiva. Look for CLPC.

Keratometry

Keratometry should be repeated and recorded on follow up visit to see if there is any effect of lens wear on the cornea.

Refraction

Do subjective refraction after about 30 minutes of lens removal. Compare the findings with the base line record. Marked changes like myopic shift or increasing astigmatism will warn against the corneal changes happening with the lenses.

Dry Eye Tests

Dry eye or dryness is the most common complaint, more so with soft lenses. Dry eye tests like Schirmer and BUT should be done after removing the lenses.

Rectify the problems on follow up visit: a review

Abnormal signs/ symptoms on follow up	*Probable cause*	*Action taken*
Pain	Tight /steep lens	Refit with flat lens (Fig. 22.2)
Fluctuating vision	Lens fit too steep or too flat	Refit
Reduced visual acuity – constant	Improper lens power Residual astigmatism Dirty lens	Correct power Refit with toric lens Replace (Fig. 22.3)
Reduced visual acuity later during the day	Hypoxia	Refit with high Dk/t
Irritation	Deposits Inadequate cleaning	Refit Improve lens care system (Fig. 22.1)
Irritation soon on insertion	Solution sensitivity improper rinsing of cleaning solution	Change sol/preservative free Improve compliance
Burning	Tight fit Hypoxia Lens dehydration	Refit – flat lens Refit with high Dk/t lens Add lubricants
Sudden pain (has been doing fine till then)	Foreign body Damaged or chipped lens	Look for and remove Replace Refit to high Dk/tRefit (Fig. 22.4)
Pain on removal	Oedema Tight lens	Refit Improve lens care system
Watering	Normal adaptive symptom Improper fitting Chipped lens/rough edge Solution sensitivity	Reassure Evaluate and refit Check and correct Look for other signs
Halos	Dirty deposited lens Optic zone smaller than pupil	Clean lens Change optic zone and diameter

Contd...

Contd...

Abnormal signs/ symptoms on follow up	*Probable cause*	*Action taken*
Frequent lens displacement	Lens is small Fit is flat	Refit
Bubbles under the lens	Lens fit is steep	Refit
Redness	Dryness Damaged lens Solution sensitivity	Add lubricants Change Change solutions
Contact lens related dryness	Dry eye Environmental condition	Better lubricating solutions Advice/ shift to FRP
Giant papillary conjunctivitis	Deposits	FRP Medical intervention
Neovascularization	Hypoxia	Refit with high Dk/t
Change in refraction	Pathological Edema Corneal distortion	Change to new power Refit with better fit/Dk/t Refit with new lens

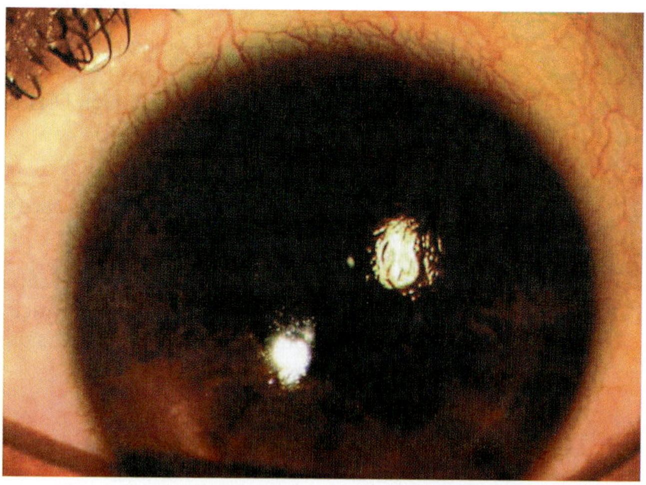

Fig. 22.1: Lens surface with deposits

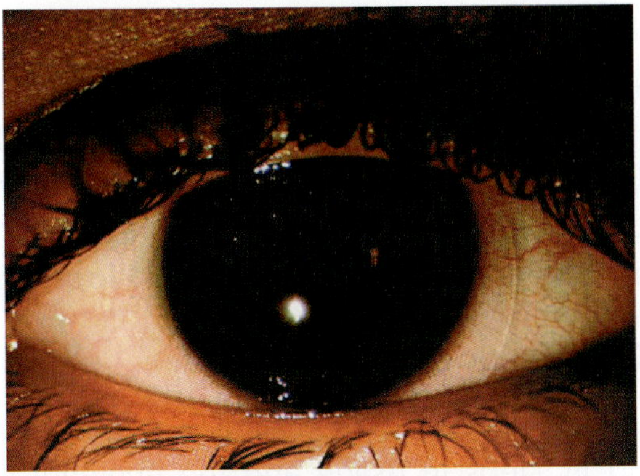

Fig. 22.2: Red eye with soft lens

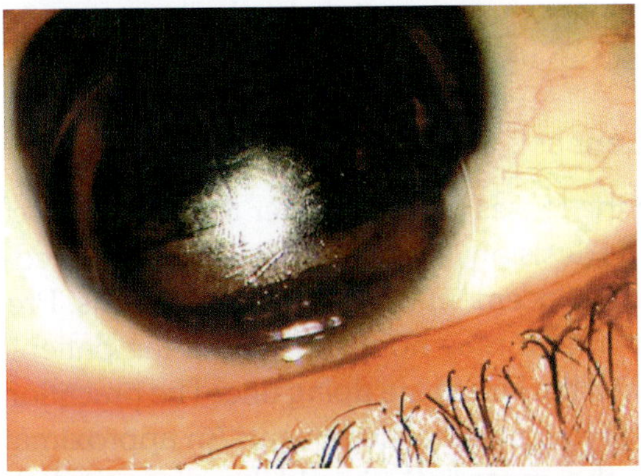

Fig. 22.3: Scratches with poor wettability

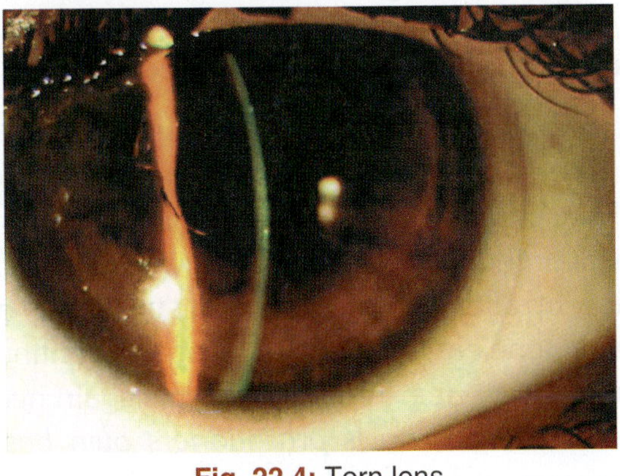

Fig. 22.4: Torn lens

"Successful" Contact Lens Wearer

The patient is said to be wearing lenses successfully if he can tolerate lenses for at least 12 hours during the day. The eye is comfortable at the end of the day. There is no redness and discomfort. The vision is also good through out the day. The patient can " ***see good***", "***feel good***" *and* "***looks good".***

Improve Compliance

After revising the lens handling, insertion and removal, use of solution and its steps in usage and the hygiene, repeat the instructions orally or in written format. Display posters and messages to improve and reinforce the important instructions during follow up visits.

Replace Lenses

To change the lenses before or after the problem occurs is the practitioner's decision. It is wiser to stress on the need of change and regular replacement to avoid complications. Prevention is better than cure. It may not be easier for the patient to accept replacement if the lenses are doing fine. The practitioner should have the skill to convince the patient. An approximate lens life (based on the material) should be discussed during the dispensing. This way the patient will not feel cheated.

Recommendations—Follow Up Schedule

Follow up appointments are usually every 6 months.
It depends upon the type of the lens material and the wearing modality. The condition of the eye is also important in deciding when the patient should visit next for follow up. Perfectly healthy eye can follow up after a longer gap and an unhealthy eye should get the review done early. Extended wear and continuous wear calls for quick follow-ups. Pediatric patients again need regular assessments. *The decision is practitioners own based on an individual wearer and cannot be guided by books.*

Next Follow Up Date

Contact lens patients are notorious for believing that regular visits are unnecessary as long as their lenses are doing fine, they are comfortable and can see well. Practitioners need to ensure that, the patient understands the need for routine ongoing after care. Schedule his next appointment before he leaves the clinic.

Comprehensive after care is an essential part of contact lens practice, irrespective of patient's symptoms.

23 Contact Lens Manufacturing and Verification

All contact lens manufacturing processes start with the polymerization of the monomer and preparation of the lens material. In some cases the pure material is then shaped in rods and cut into buttons.

There are 3 basic methods of manufacturing contact lenses:
1. Lathe cutting
2. Spin casting
3. Cast molding

LATHE CUTTING (Fig. 23.1)

A hard dry button of the contact lens polymer is ground on the lathe machine. The front, back and peripheral curves are cut from the button according to the specifications. Nowadays computerized lathe machines are available which cut the intermediate and peripheral curves along with the edge designs.

The cut lens is then removed from the lathe and polished to make the surface smooth and to have a clear optics.

This process can be used for all rigid and soft lenses.

For soft lenses the lathe cut lens undergoes the next step of hydration before packing.

Hydration of Soft Lenses

The lathe cut dry soft lens polymer is immersed in saline and hydrated. This transforms the lens into a soft and flexible lens. The calculations for cutting the lens parameters are precalculated so that the exact curvatures and power is obtained after hydration.

Advantages

Custom designs for an individual patient can be made

Disadvantages

- It is time consuming and labor intensive process
- Production is possible in low quantities only
- Ultra thin designs are difficult to achieve by this process.
- Reproducibility is a problem at times.

SPIN CASTING

OttoWichterle invented the first method used for making soft lenses in 1951 by spin casting. This process is still widely used to manufacture soft lenses.

In this process a liquid polymer is injected into a spinning mold. The spinning mould creates a lens design where the front

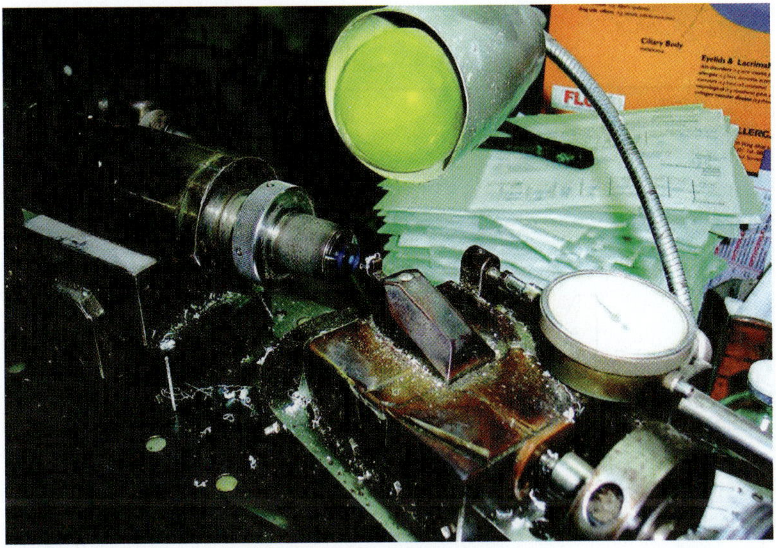

Fig. 23.1: Lathe process

surface is determined by the curvature of the mold and the back surface depends upon the speed of the spinning mold, temperature, gravity, surface tension, amount of liquid polymer and the centrifugal force (Fig. 23.2A).

Curing

The second step is curing. Where the liquid polymer is transformed into a solid state by treating the lens material by heat or ultraviolet radiation. This solid lens is then hydrated in saline the same way as done for lathe cut lens (Fig. 23.2B).

Advantages

- Lenses can be produced in large quantities
- They can be easily reproduced
- The surface obtained is aspheric
- It produces thin and comfortable edge designs
- It is inexpensive.

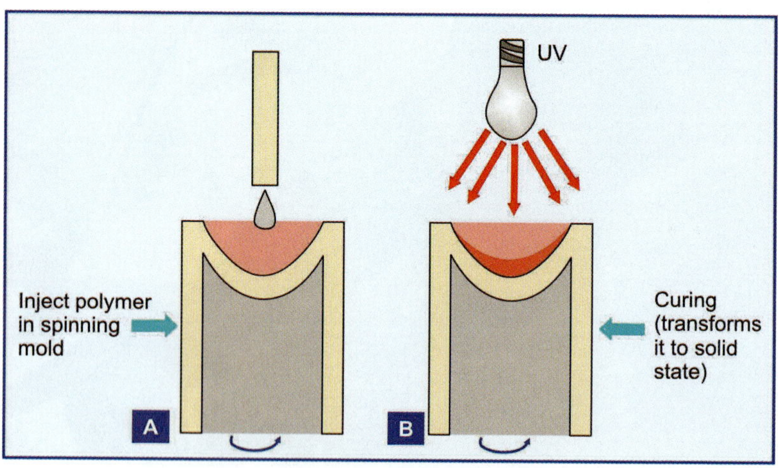

Fig. 23.2: Spin cast

Disadvantages

Only limited parameters or designs are possible by this method.

CAST MOLDING

In this process the liquid polymer is poured in the concave mold. The convex mold is then clamped over the concave mold. The polymer is then cured by ultraviolet radiation. The dry state of the lens is then removed and hydrated (Fig. 23.3).

For each design a separate kind of mold is required. The concave surface determines the front surface and the convex mold creates a back surface. This process now manufactures most of the disposable lenses.

The above process has the following advantages:

- It is fast and less labor intensive
- It is cost effective
- Parameters of lenses can be duplicated exactly
- High volumes can be produced
- Complex designs are possible.

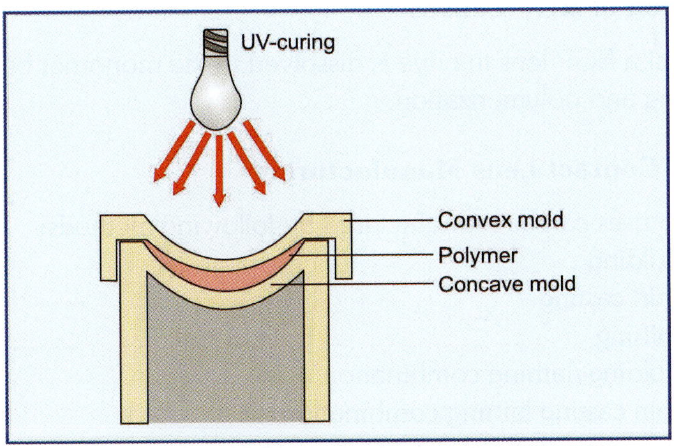

Fig. 23.3: Cast molding

Disadvantages

- Custom made lenses cannot be made by this process
- It requires a large manufacturing unit and the initial cost is more
- Not all materials are suitable for molding.

Quality Assurance and Inspection

This is an important step and the inspection is performed of every lens prior to packaging and distribution.

Sterilization

The lenses are sterilized before dispensing. The method mostly employed is autoclaving. The lenses are autoclaved at a temperature of 124 degrees celsius for at least 20 minutes.

RGP Manufacturing

RGP lenses are manufacture by 2 methods:

- Lathing—used commonly
- Molding—recently adapted technique.

Tinting of RGP Lenses

To tint a RGP lens the dye is dissolved in the monomer before mixing and polymerization.

Soft Contact Lens Manufacturing

Soft lenses can be manufactured by following methods:

- Molding
- Spin casting
- Lathing
- Molding /lathing combination
- Spin casting lathing combination
- Molding—stabilized soft technique.

Molding /lathing combination: Usually the back surface is molded and the front surface is lathed

Spin casting/ lathing combination: Usually the front surface is spin cast and the back surface is lathed

Stabilized soft molding: A space taking inert diluent is included in the mix of monomers during polymerization. This diluent is replaced by water later. The final product thus achieved thus undergoes minimal change on hydration and provided high quality optics and surface finish.

CONTACT LENS VERIFICATION

The contact lens once ordered should be verified before dispensing. Though the laboratories try to maintain standards, yet there are possibilities and errors, which are due to the manufacturing. A faulty lens will not conform to the design specially ordered.

Simple equipments that can be a part of the contact lens clinic can verify the parameters. Some parameters need sophisticated equipments, which can be done in the laboratories.

The following parameters, which need to be verified, are:

1. Base curve
2. Power
3. Diameter
4. Central thickness
5. Surface quality
6. Edge
7. Blend
8. Material

Base Curve

- Radiuscope
- Keratometer

Radiuscope (Fig. 23.4)

The Radiuscope is the most commonly used instrument in the laboratory to verify the base curve.

It is based on the *Drysdale's principle.* If an object is placed at the radius of curvature of the curved surface, the real image created by the instrument acts as an object and will form an image at the second focal point. The real image is formed at the first focal plane and the virtual image is formed at the second focal plane, both being the centre of curvature of the lens.

The lens RGP (in dry state- soaked 24 hrs before) and the soft lens (in wet cell with 0.9% saline) is kept with concave side up on the lens mount. The first focal plane mires are focused, the reading is set at zero at this position. The dial is further moved

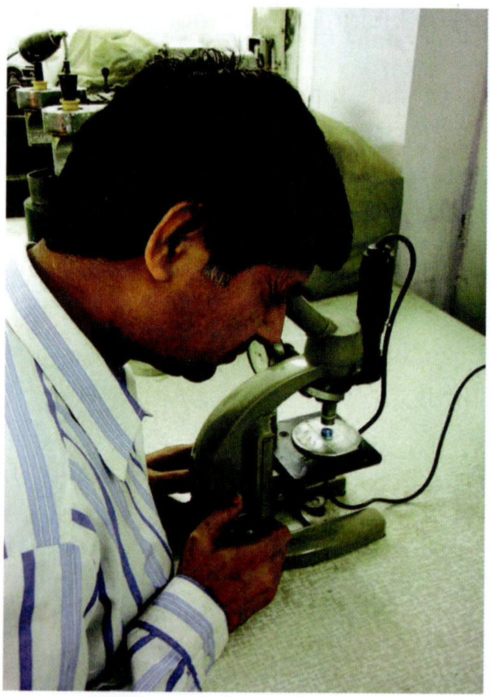

Fig. 23.4: Radiuscope

to focus the second set of mires, which is the second focal point. The distance between the two focal points measures the radius of curvature, which is read from the dial.

In case of a toric lens the mires will have two set of lines perpendicular to each other, which will be focused separately. A warped lens will show no definite base curve.

The **Keratometer** can also be used to verify the base curve, though not very accurate. The set up is modified with the lens holder and a mirror attachment. The lens is held with the help of this holder and the readings taken same ways the Keratometer is used.

POWER VERIFICATION

Focimeter/Lensometer (Figs 23.5 and 23.6)

This instrument is used exactly as for the spectacle lens. The contact lens is cleaned first and then centered concave side down on the focimeter stop. Read the values on the drum. The prism can also be measured the same way as in spectacle lenses. The lens power should be within +/– 0.25 D of the power ordered.

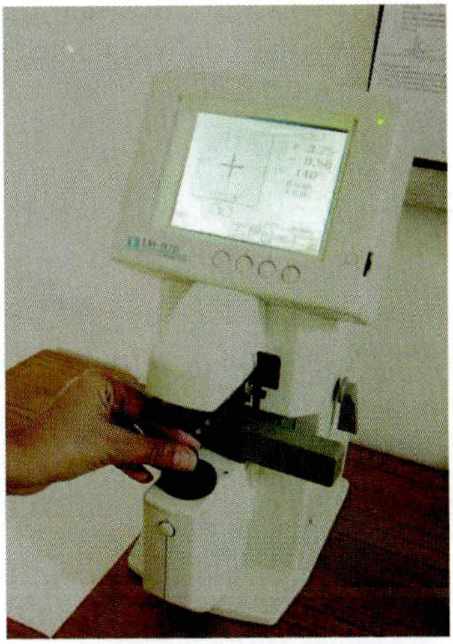

Fig. 23.5: Lensometer

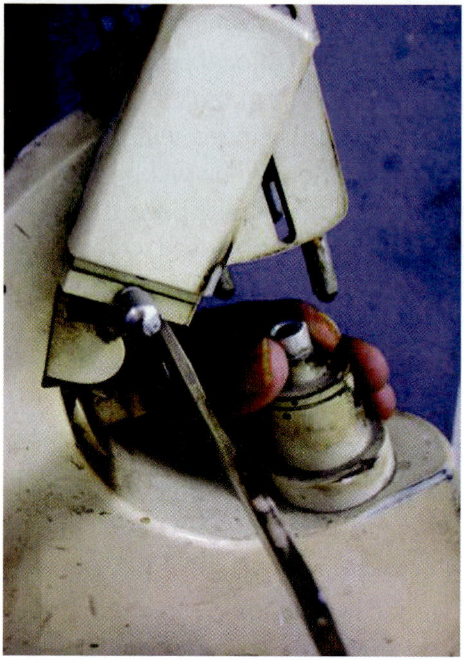

Fig. 23.6: Lens on focimeter

In case of toric lenses two line focuses will be obtained. The two principal meridians are noted and then transposed to read the spherical and the cylindrical values.

Diameter

The V sought gauge (Fig. 23.7) or the measuring loupe can verify the diameter of the RGP lens. The lens is made to slide across the V slought and allowed to fall into the proper position by its own weight. Note the reading in millimeter corresponding on the scale. While measuring ensure that the:

- Lens is dry
- Take care not to exercise any force while inserting the lens into the gauge
- Check in two meridians for roundness
- The tolerance limit is +/–0.05 mm.

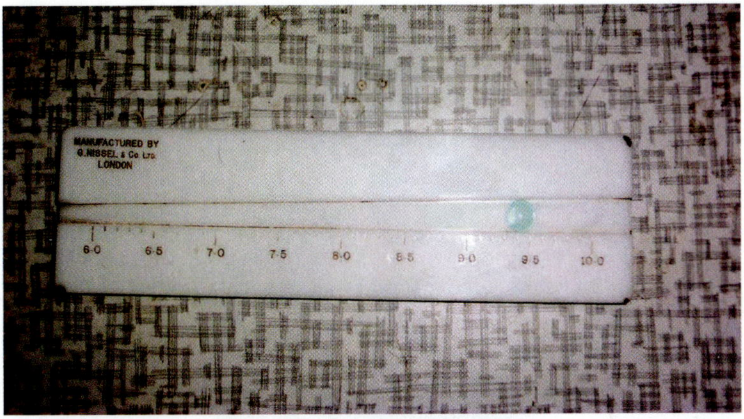

Fig. 23.7: V slought gauge

The *measuring magnifier*—the lens is held across the magnifier and the scale reading of the diameter are correspondingly read. This also serves the dual purpose of measuring the diameter and the width of the peripheral and the optic zone.

The *soft lens analyzer* or the projection devices in wet state can also measure the soft lens diameter.

Central Thickness

The **thickness gauge or the dial gauge** is the most useful device for measuring central thickness (Fig. 23.8).

The lens is placed convex side down on its base. A spring plunger tip is released until it touches the lens. The thickness is read directly on the gauge. Ensure the zero error before hand.

Surface Quality

Various types of projection devices available can measure the surface quality and the edge profile. The **projection analyzer** can also be used to measure the optic zone diameter and the peripheral curves width.

The surface can also be inspected by use of slit lamp. Use monochromatic light and inspect the lens.

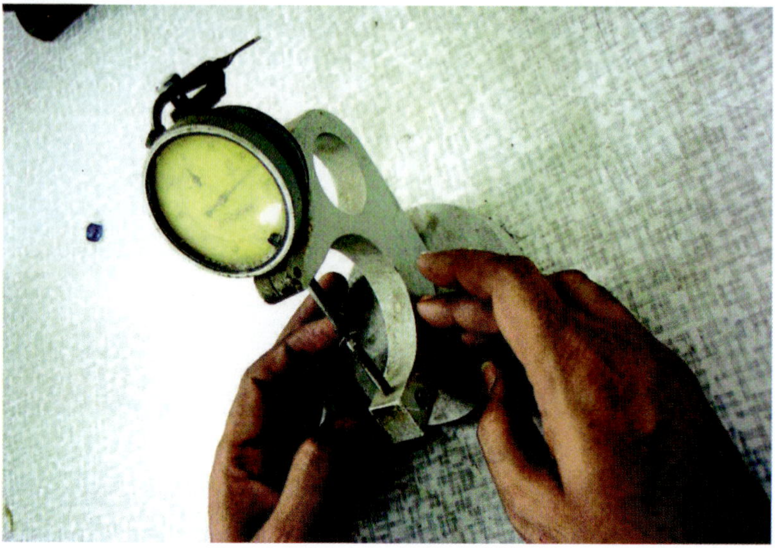

Fig. 23.8: Thickness dial

Blend and Edge Shape (Fig. 23.9)

The **projection analyzer or the magnifying loupe** is used to examine the transition zones of the peripheral curves.

Edge is most important for the comfort of the RGP lens. The faulty lens can create problems, so it is essential to inspect the lens edge of an uncomfortable lens. The lens can be held; with the help of a holder, and the image of the lens edge can be created on the wall by holding the lens in the slit-lamp illumination. As discussed earlier the round edge is the most comfortable one.

Material

All Rigid materials look same but have a fixed specific gravity. The material can be verified by testing its specific gravity. Different solutions bottles with known specific gravity are needed. The lens is dipped in the bottles one by one. The specific gravity can be calculated if it floats or sinks in the known specific gravity.

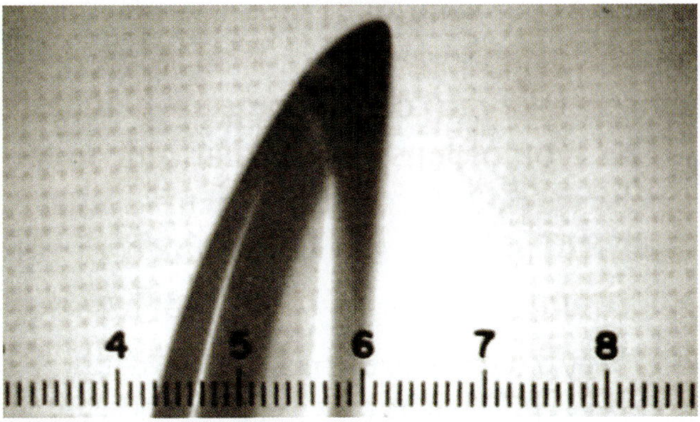

Fig. 23.9: Edge examination with magnifier

Verification of Parameters—Summary

- Base curve—Radiuscope
- Diameter—V slought gauge
- Power—Lensometer
- Central thickness—Dial gauge
- Peripheral curves/width/blend—Projection analyzer or magnifying loupe
- Material—Specific gravity test.

24 Rigid Contact Lens Modification

Seldom, it may be necessary that rigid lens needs to be modified before dispensing. This may have happened because one may have erred in estimating the final parameters for an eye. Rather than reordering the lens and loosing on the profits one can do or get some small modifications on the same lens.

This can be even faster if the equipment is available in the office.

This chapter will guide regarding the methods of modifications that can be done by equipments in the laboratory.

It is important for the practitioner to understand the possible modifications, which can be done before delivery of the lens in case needed.

The following is the list of possible adjustments that can be made on the lens:

1. Reducing overall diameter
2. Blending transition zones
3. Flattening intermediate curves
4. Reducing optic zone diameter
5. Adding minus power
6. Adding plus power?
7. Removing scratches
8. Polishing and refinishing the lens.

It is clear from the above list that one can modify the lens to produce a flat or loose fit or flatten the peripheral curves. Power, also is safer to add minus than plus.

Thus, it is safer to err towards a steeper fitting or lesser minus power.

Polishing the Lens Surface (Fig. 24.1)

i. Use The polishing compound like XPAL
ii. To polish the **front surface**—center the lens, convex side outside, with the suction cup
iii. Use the flat sponge tool
iv. Hold the rotating spindle at 45 degrees on the outer side of the sponge tool and rotate in the opposite direction.
v. Keep applying the polish liberally
vi. Depress the lens in the sponge for 10 to 15 seconds, with minimal pressure
vii. Polish the center holding the sponge perpendicular at the center
viii. Inspect every 10 seconds for the surface quality
ix. To polish the **concave surface** use a cone shaped sponge tool and hold the lens concave side out with the suction

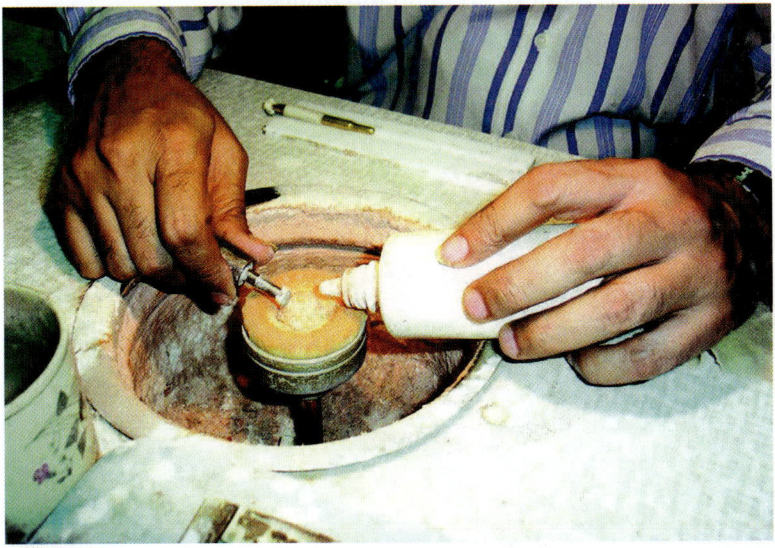

Fig. 24.1: Polishing the lens surface

cup. Hold the lens perpendicular and depress with minimal pressure.

Adding the Power (Fig. 24.2)

It is easier to *add minus power* without spoiling the optics. The maximum of one diopter can be added to a lens.

i. Use a moistened flat sponge tool
ii. Hold the lens with the suction cup, approximately 2.5 cm from the edge of the lens
iii. Apply minimal pressure and rotate in direction opposite to the rotating handle
iv. Check power every 10 to 15 seconds
v. This step is similar to polishing, that means polishing always adds some amount of minus power
vi. *Adding plus power:* The lens has to be held perpendicular exactly in the center, applying pressure so that the periphery is polished. This makes the front surface more convex, hence adds plus power. Only 0.25 to 0.50 plus power can be added without spoiling the optics.

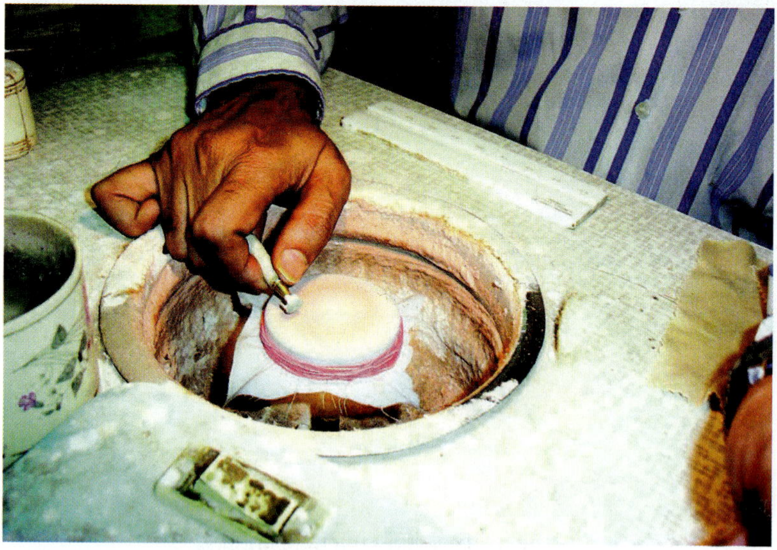

Fig. 24.2: Adding the power

Reducing the Overall Diameter (Fig. 24.3)

i. Use a cut down stone tool, use emery, stone or diamond polish
ii. Hold the lens concave side out with the suction cup
iii. Bring the lens slowly down, perpendicular to the rotating cut down stone tool
iv. With light pressure, place the lens in the tool.
v. Check the diameter regularly till the target is reached.

Flattening the Peripheral Curves

i. Use a radius stool and apply adhesive tape over it. Select the tool depending upon the curvature desired. Take the tool 0.2 mm lesser than the desired curvature (this is done to compensate for the adhesive thickness).
Suppose 10.0 mm curvature is desired, select 9.8 mm tool.
ii. Hold the lens on the spindle handle or a suction cup, with concave side outside.

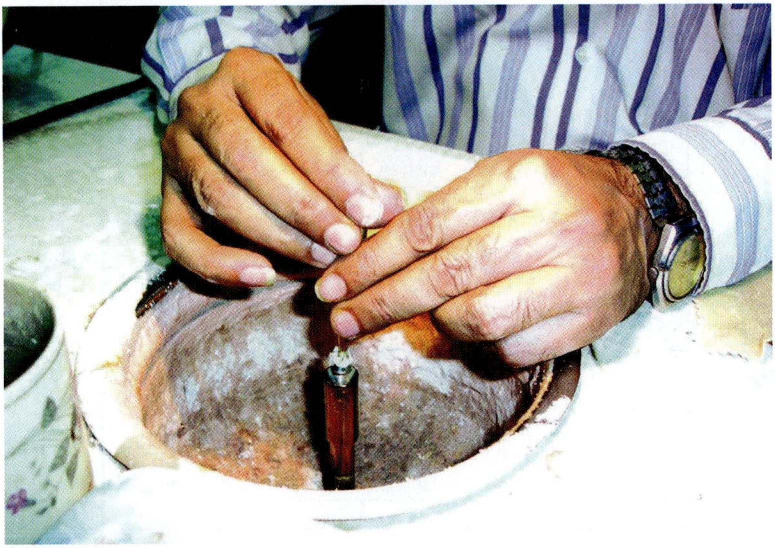

Fig. 24.3: Reducing the overall diameter

iii. With the spinner handle, center the lens on the spinner tool and hold 45 to 60 degrees off the center of the radius tool.
iv. Apply polish, liberally throughout the procedure.
v. Regularly monitor the curves by the eye loupe

Flatten PC

Blending of the Junctions (Fig. 24.4)

i. Select a tool with a radius half way between the two adjacent curves.
ii. Cover the tool with a soft flannel cloth.
iii. Repeat the same procedure like as done in adjusting the peripheral curves.
iv. Monitor at intervals so that the blending is not too heavy.

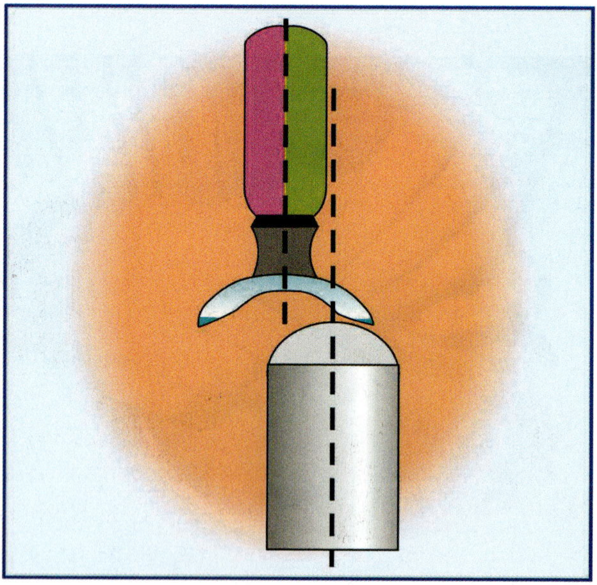

Fig. 24.4: Blending junctions

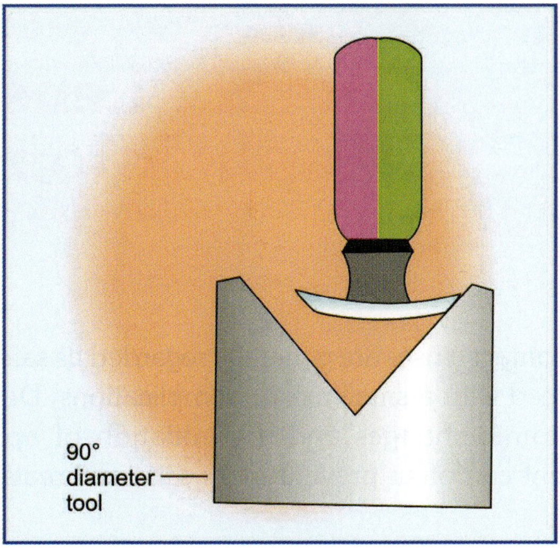

Fig. 24.5: Modifying the edge

Edge Modification (Fig. 24.5)

i. Use the 90 degrees conic tool and adhesive tape over it.
ii. Holding the lens with the suction cup, convex side outside, creates an anterior bevel.
iii. Apply polish liberally throughout.
iv. Place the lens in the cone gently, so that it cuts the edge smoothly.
v. Check the edge thickness every 10 seconds, till desired is achieved.
vi. Polish the edge smooth, with the flat sponge tool later. To alter the lens shape and rounding off, use the flat sponge tool only. Hold the lens with the rotating spinner, concave side out and smoothen the inner side.

25 Contact Lens Complications

Although contact lenses are generally regarded as safe, yet they are associated with a small risk or complications. Detection of these anatomic changes and the initiation of appropriate management can often prevent more serious threats of vision loss.

Why do Complications Occur?

As such, lenses do not cause any complications. They usually happen because of

- **Mechanical reasons**—when the lens fitting is not proper or the quality of the lens may be poor.
- **Physiological reasons**—when the oxygen requirement of the cornea is physiologically compromised thus leading to hypoxic reactions of the cornea.
- **Environmental reasons**
- **Noncompliance**—when it happens due to the neglect of the patient in following proper care and maintenance instructions, ignoring symptoms, over wearing of lenses, sharing of lenses and solutions, etc.

These are the reasons when we assume that the practitioner has made no error. Where as, very often, one may come across contact lens related complications due to lack of knowledge of the practitioner.

It is moral responsibility of the practitioner to be able to at least detect them and provide or refer, for suitable management to the ophthalmologist.

A review of some of the common contact lens complications will be presented in this chapter. These complications will be discussed on the basis if etiology (cause), symptom (indication or disorder as noticed by the patient), sign (indications as noticed by the practitioner).

Corneal Ulcer Infected— (Serious Complication) (Fig. 25.1)

Infected corneal ulcers are the most serious complication associated with contact lens wear. An ulcer is defined, as the full thickness epithelial loss with stromal necrosis and inflammation, may be central or paracentral.

Etiology

It is thought that hypoxia leads to reduction in ability of the eye to resist invading organism. The most important organisms leading to serious infections are *Pseudomonas aeruginosa* and *Acanthamoeba*.

The infection can be passed on from patient's contaminated hands, lens case, solution or may be an improperly disinfected lens.

The incidence of ulcers is maximum with extended wear soft lenses (21 in 10,000), which reduces to, 4 in 10,000 with soft lenses and, 1 in 10, 000 with RGP lenses.

That is again related to hypoxia, which is most likely with extended wear soft lenses.

Acanthamoeba is an uncommon but an infection that causes severe ocular damage. The condition was first reported in 1973. It is suspected more in soft lens wearers particularly those who use home made saline and tap water.

Symptoms

- Foreign body sensation to extreme pain
- Redness

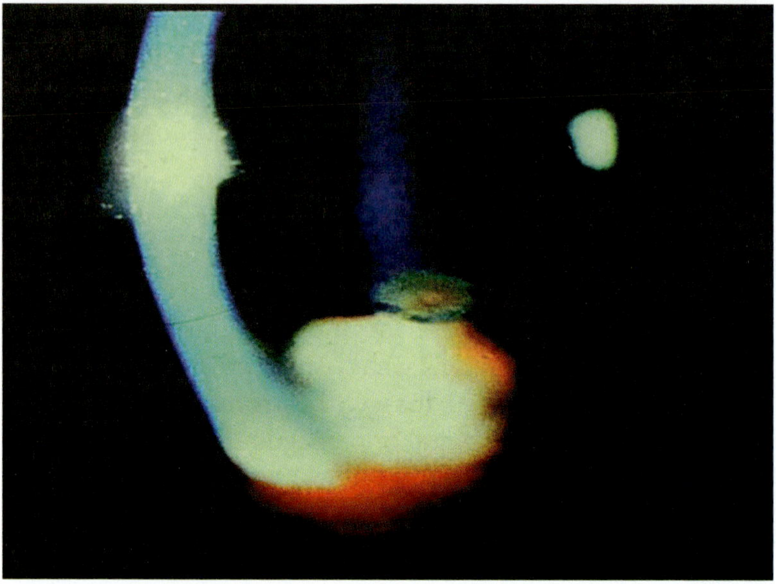

Fig. 25.1: Corneal ulcer

- Mucoid discharge (bacterial), watery (viral), purulent to watery (fungal)
- Photophobia
- Reduced visual acuity if ulcer is in pupillary area.

Signs

- Intense redness, generally diffused but can be localized
- Usually unilateral
- Opaque white area in the cornea
- Infiltrates
- Lid edema
- May be associated with anterior chamber flare.

Management

- Remove lenses immediately
- Refer for medical treatment—includes corneal scraping for smear and culture prior to treatment, start broad spectrum antibiotic therapy

- No lens wear for 2- 3 months
- Refit with new lens and reinsure compliance.

Prevention

In the prevention of ulcer the patient and the practitioner play a very important role. One can reduce such sight-threatening complications if:

- Patient/practitioner is aware of the warning signs
- He does not sleep with the lenses (unless recommended)
- Stress on proper hygiene and compliance
- Home made saline and tap water have a higher risk of infection
- Regular follow-ups even if there is no complaint.

CLPU—Contact Lens Peripheral Ulcer

This is a round full thickness epithelial loss with *inflamed* base, *typically in corneal periphery,* which results in scar.

They are generally small ulcers less than 1 mm in diameter. They are also not associated with any sign of anterior chamber flare and stain with fluorescein dye.

Corneal Neovascularization (Fig. 25.2)

It is the growth of the limbal blood vessels into the cornea. The vessel extension beyond translucent limbal zone is recorded in millimeters. Small amounts 1 to 2 mm are common, more than 2 mm is a warning sign. If this progresses into the visual axis it can lead to vision loss. It may be superficial deep, superficial or all around 360 degrees into the cornea.

Etiology

The most common reason is hypoxia. Others include solution sensitivity, or mechanical effects like poor fit or damaged lens.

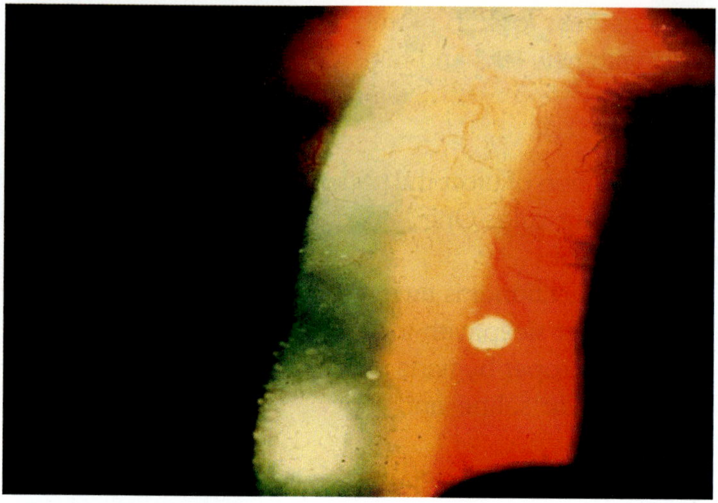

Fig. 25.2: Neovascularization

Symptoms

- Asymptomatic
- Vision effected if vessel growth is over pupil.

Signs

- Vessel growth seen around limbus
- It may be looped if inactive or branching if active.

Management

- Discontinue wear till vessels are emptied of blood
- Refit with higher oxygen permeable lens
- Advice daily wear mode only
- Discontinue wear permanently if severe neovascularization.

Prevention

- Regular follow-ups and examination
- Refit with better oxygen transmissibility lenses if NVE observed.

Corneal Edema—Striae and Folds (Figs 25.3 and 25.4)

Edema is the swelling of the cornea due to increased accumulation of the fluid in the stroma. Edema leads to separation of collagen fibrils and if increases lead to corneal haze.

Chronic levels of corneal edema, even if low, result in adverse effects on functioning of the cornea.

Symptoms

- Patient is symptomatic only if the corneal edema is greater than 20%
- Higher levels cause glare, haloes around light and decreased acuity.

Signs

Observe in optical section of the cornea
- Striae—fine grayish white vertical lines mostly in the posterior stroma (One striae signifies 5% edema)
- Folds—fine grey lines, buckling of the posterior cornea (One fold signifies 8% edema)
- Each additional striae or fold indicates 1% more edema.
- Loss of corneal transparency if edema is more than 20%.

Management

- Edema resolves in around 3 hours after removal of lenses
- Chronic edema may take one week to resolve
- Refit with higher oxygen transmissibility lens
- Decrease wearing time.

Precautions

- Commonly found in extended wear
- Refit when warning signs are first seen
- High plus powers should be carefully followed, as central thickness is more.

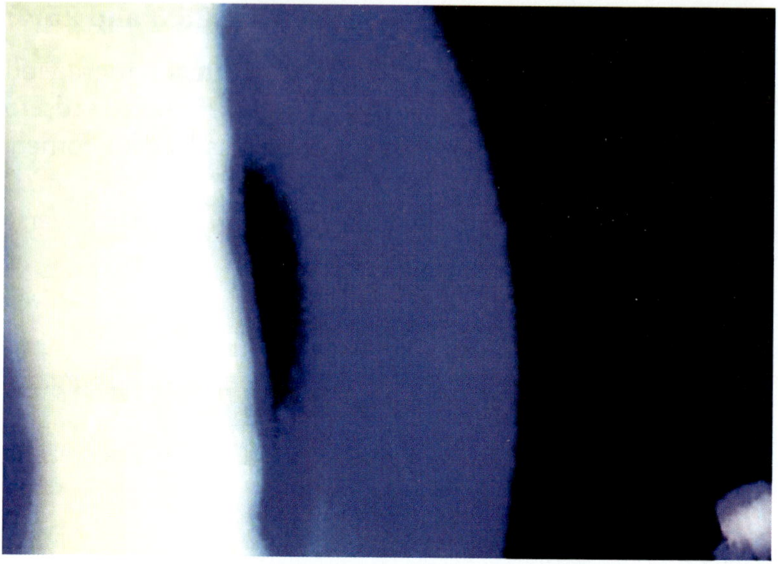

Fig. 25.3: Corneal striae

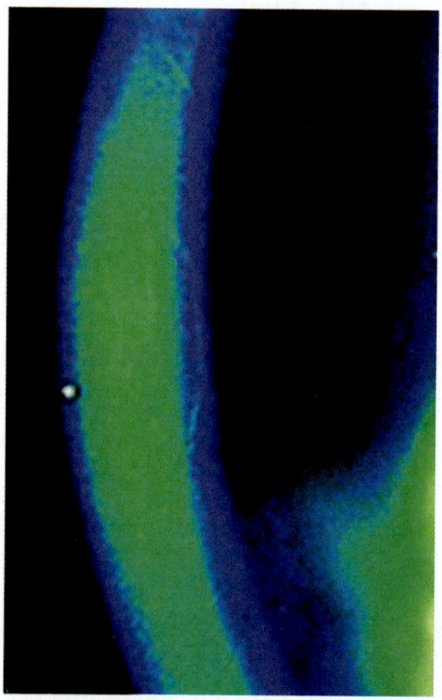

Fig. 25.4: Striae folds

Inflammatory Ocular Responses

Infiltrates (Figs 25.5 and 25.6)

Infiltrates means the infiltration of the cornea with aggregates of the inflammatory cells such as neutrophils, macrophages, and lymphocytes. This happens as an inflammatory response to the stimuli. They are white opacities observed epithelial, subepithelial or stromal depending upon the layer of the cornea.

Etiology

They occur in conjunction with acute red eye, corneal ulcer or infection, localized trauma, solution sensitivity and prolonged hypoxia. The incidence of infiltrates is more in soft lenses used for extended wear.

Symptoms

- May be asymptomatic, depends upon severity
- Photophobia
- Foreign body sensation
- Watering
- Redness or pain
- Depending upon the etiology.

Signs

- White opacities most frequently seen 2 -3 mm from limbus
- May be focal or diffuse.

Management

- Discontinue lens wear
- Treat the underlying etiology by determining the cause.

Prevention

- Prevent recurrence based on the etiology
- Refit with RGP if reoccurs with soft lenses.

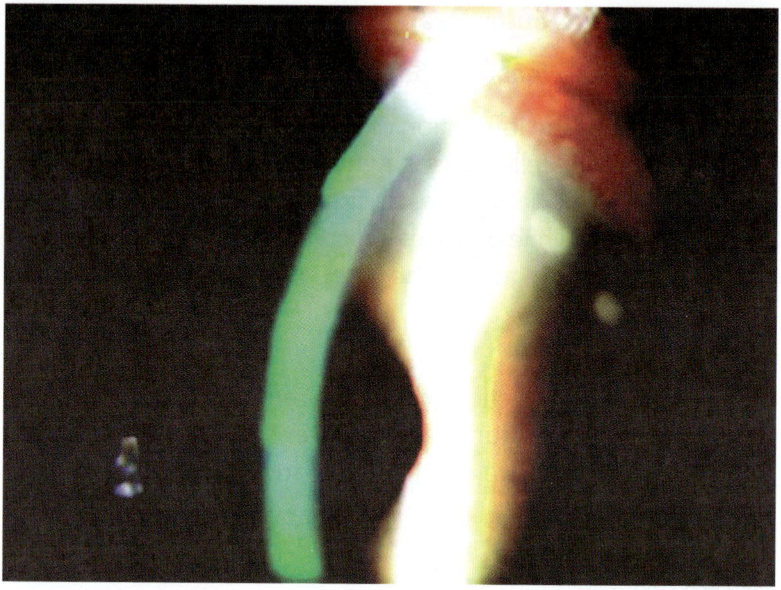

Fig. 25.5: Infiltrate—focal (*Courtsey:* IACLE)

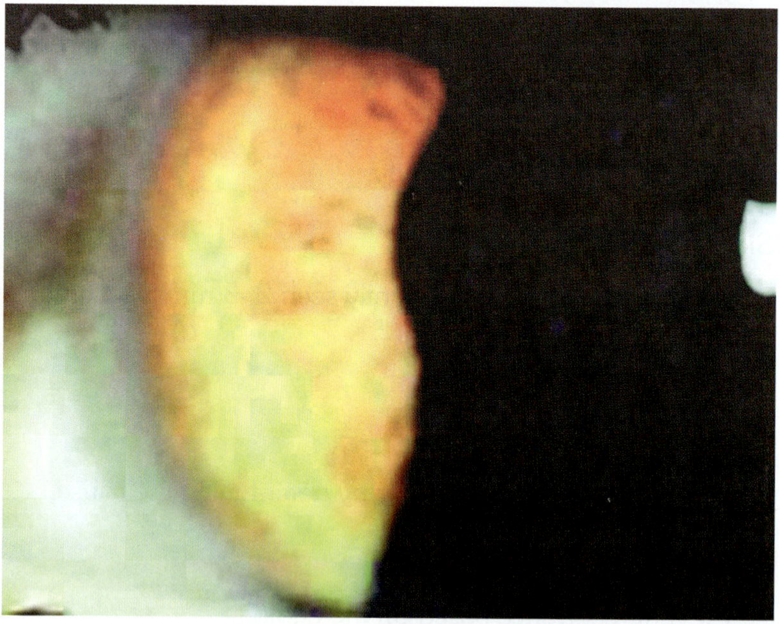

Fig. 25.6: Infiltrate—diffuse (*Courtsey:* IACLE)

CLARE—Contact Lens Acute Red Eye (Fig. 25.7)

It is a serious inflammatory response reaction reported frequently with extended wear lenses.

Etiology

Red eye is an inflammatory response that can be from hypoxia to contamination to an ill-fitting lens.

Symptoms

- This is typically seen in extended wear patients who wake up with painful red eye in the morning
- It may be associated with watering and photophobia
- Vision is affected if it is severe.

Signs

- Associated with infiltrates
- Redness
- Usually unilateral.

Management

- Discontinue lens wear
- Refer for medical intervention – antimicrobial therapy if due to infection
- Resume lens wear after 2 weeks.

Prevention

- Avoid extended wear
- Check fitting particularly avoid steep fitting
- Proper hygiene
- Frequent replacement
- Warn patient of the warning signs.

Contact Lens-induced Papillary Conjunctivitis—CLPC (Giant Papillary Conjunctivitis) (Figs 25.8 and 25.9)

CLPC is the inflammatory response of the upper tarsal conjunctiva. The smooth conjunctiva becomes rough, bumpy

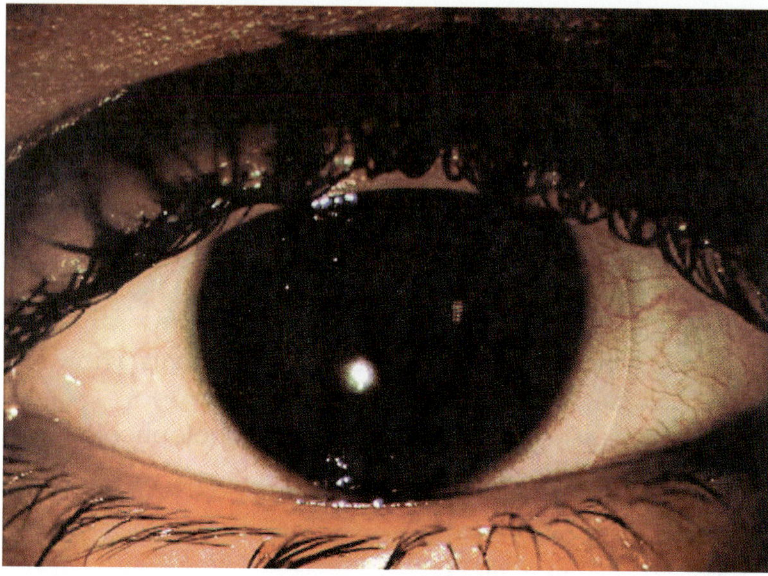

Fig. 25.7: CLARE

and uneven. The condition progresses from mild to severe stage if the predisposing factor is not removed. GPC is one of the major reasons for lens dropouts. Its incidence reduces remarkably if the lenses are replaced frequently. CLPC is less likely to occur with RGP lenses.

Etiology

This is an inflammatory response that is induced by the deposits or any mechanical interaction between lid and lens.

Symptoms

- Depends upon the grade and severity
- Stage 1 is preclinical and patient is asymptomatic
- Itchiness
- Mucous strands
- Lens intolerance/reduced wearing time
- Excess lens movement.

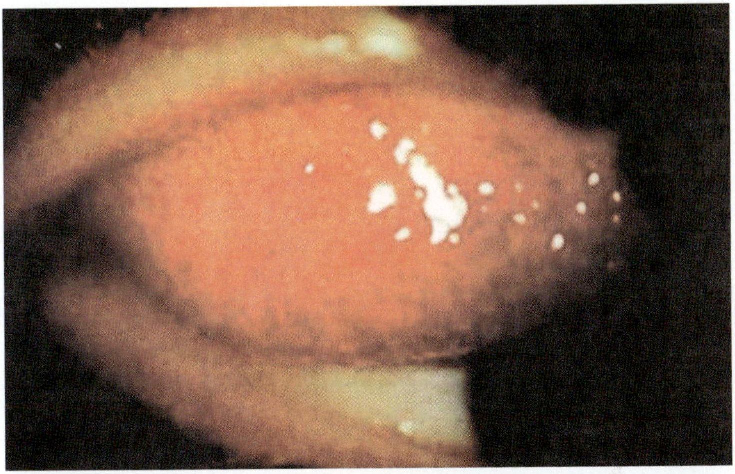

Fig. 25.8: CLPC

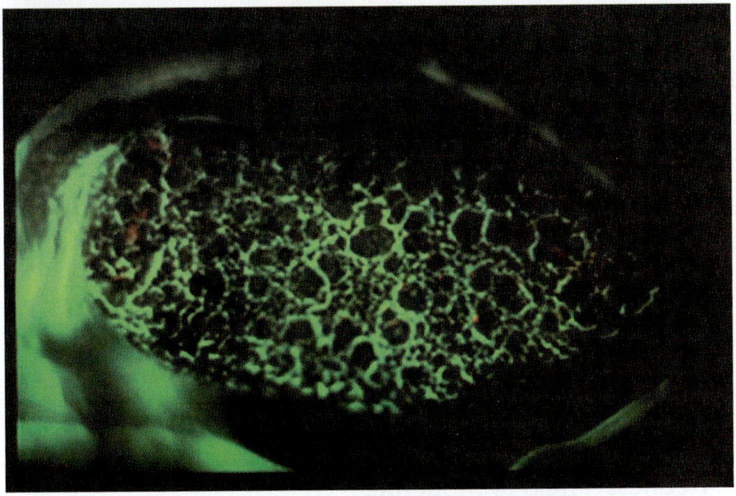

Fig. 25.9: CLPC—stained with fluorescein

Signs

- Enlarged papillae—bumpy upper lid on eversion
- Lid redness
- Mucus strands
- Lens moves more.

Management

- Discontinue lens wear till GPC subside—may be one or two months
- Shift patient to FRP
- No extended wear
- Find the cause and treat.

Prevention

- Early detection by regular follow-ups
- Frequent replacement program
- Enzyme treatment to reduce deposits.

Sensitivity to Solutions

The preservatives in the solutions can cause immediate allergic reactions or delayed hypersensitivity reactions. The patient develops an inflammatory reaction.

Symptoms

- Reduced tolerance to lenses
- Gritty sensation
- Dryness
- Itching.

Signs

- Superficial corneal damage
- Redness—mild to moderate
- Infiltrates (may be)
- Papillae.

Management

- Cease use of preserved solutions
- Try other preservative group

- Shift patient to unpreserved unit doze solutions with thermal disinfection or peroxide system of disinfection
- FRP—frequent replacement program.

Epithelial or Subepithelial Corneal Staining (Figs 25.10A and B)

Corneal staining can be identified with fluorescein dye. Any damage to the cornea can be seen as green stain seen with slit lamp and cobalt blue light. With all aberrations the lens wear should be ceased. Superficial epithelial damage will heal within 24 hours. Deeper ones diffused into the stroma may take 2 to 7 days.

Staining can be of various types and typically diagnostic of several complications. It should be routine to instill fluorescein in the eye and examine for any corneal staining.

Corneal staining may be seen in—corneal aberrations, superficial punctuate keratitis, 3 and 9 o'clock staining, arcuate defects or dry eye.

Corneal Aberrations

They occur because of some mechanical trauma to the eye. This may be due to fingernail, a foreign body under the lens or mechanical pressure due to a tight or flat fit. These aberrations are more commonly found in RGP lenses. With an aberration on the eye the patient is at risk to microbes that can penetrate the cornea easily. It is also seen that aberrations infected with pseudomonas lead to serious corneal ulcers.

Symptoms

- The patient is uncomfortable
- Pain
- Watering
- Intolerance to lens wear.

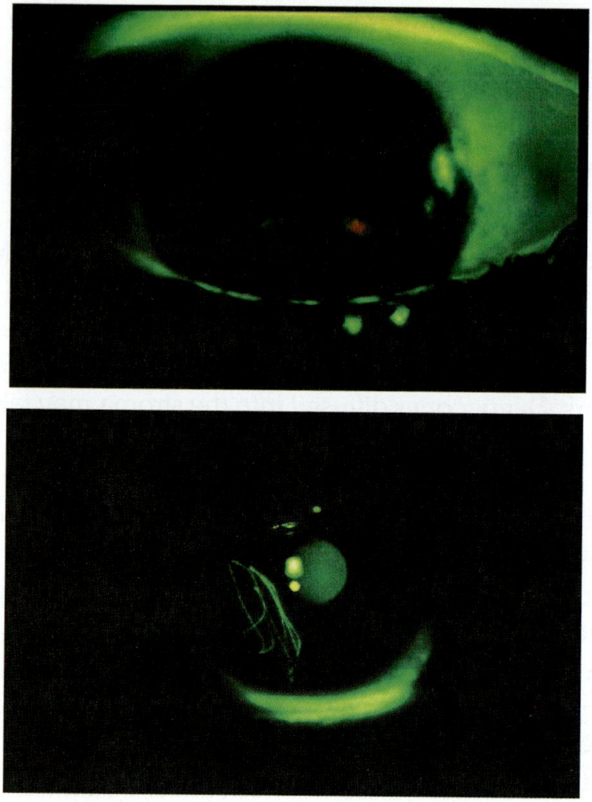

Figs 25.10A and B: Corneal aberration (*Courtsey:* IACLE)

Management

- Discontinue wear till aberration heals
- Treat the cause
- Prevent chances of infection
- Refit if improper lens.

Toxic Staining (Fig. 25.11)

Solution preservatives can cause toxic reactions. A typical diffuse superficial punctuate staining all over the cornea can be seen with the slit-lamp.

Symptoms

- Discomfort
- Burning and stinging sensation soon on insertion of lens.

Signs

- Conjunctival redness
- SPK—superficial punctuate keratitis.

Management

- Change solutions
- Shift to unpreserved system of disinfection

Superficial Epithelial Arcuate Lesion—SEAL (Fig. 25.12)

Epithelial defect in arcuate pattern often at the periphery or mid-periphery, usually superior, may be seen in a tight fitting soft lens or also due to pressure of lid on the lens.

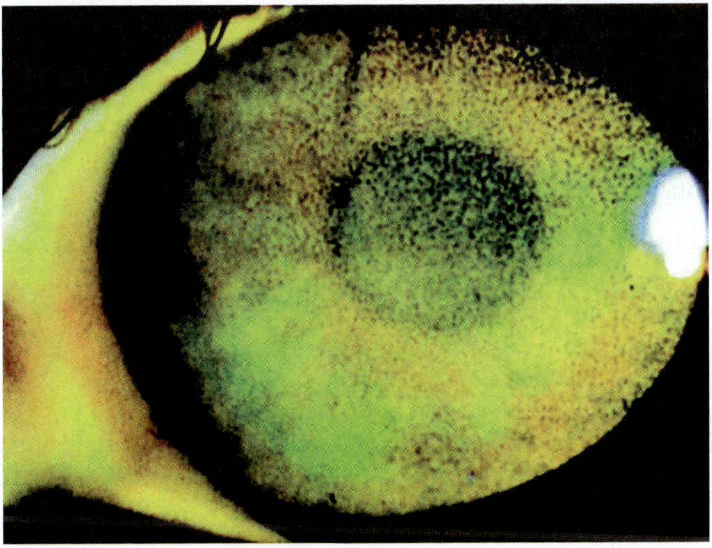

Fig. 25.11: Toxic stain

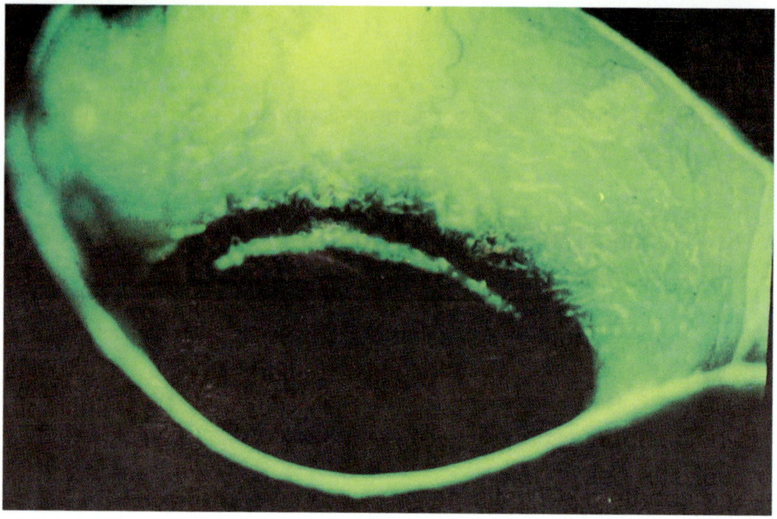

Fig. 25.12: SEAL (*Courtsey:* IACLE)

Symptoms

May be asymptomatic.

Signs

Superior arcuate shaped lesion staining with fluorescein dye.

Management

- Change to different lens type material and design
- Use a well-blended peripheral curve design
- Consider RGP.

3 and 9 o' Clock Staining (Fig. 25.13)

This condition of corneal staining is typically seen in rigid lenses. It is caused by desiccation of the cornea which occurs as a result of an interruption of tear flow or tear layer at the nasal and temporal cornea.

The disruption of the tear layer can be because of a poor edge fitting.

- A flat lens on astigmatic cornea
- A wide edge of an daily wear lens
- Low riding lens with edges touching the nasal and temporal cornea
- Poor wettability of the lens
- Narrow edge if the RGP is for extended wear mode
- This staining can also be because of patients poor tear quality. Patients who avoid blink to reduce lid interaction ultimately develop this kind of staining
- Persistent staining will lead to stromal thinning and dellen formation.

Symptoms

- Intolerance to lens wear
- Dryness.

Signs

- Typical staining at nasal and temporal cornea—the 3 and 9 o' clock position
- Redness of conjunctiva at these positions
- Infiltrates in advanced cases.

Management

- Identify the cause
- Modify the edge design
- Improve blinking
- Check tear quality
- Use in eye lubricants
- Refit with larger diameter.

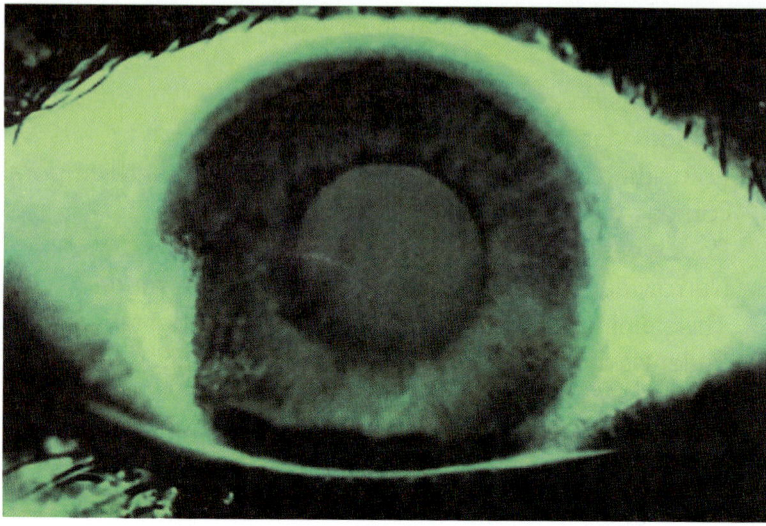

Fig. 25.13: 3 and 9 o'clock staining (*Courtsey:* IACLE)

THE ADVERSE EFFECT OF LENSES

We have discussed hypoxia and the critical levels of oxygen required by cornea to maintain its functional and structural integrity. This chapter will outline the ocular changes in different layers of the cornea that may happen with lenses *due to hypoxia, acidosis and as an inflammatory response.*

Effect on Epithelium

1. *Microcysts* : They resemble degenerated epithelial cells, which represent a delayed response to chronic epithelial hypoxia. They take an average of 2 to 3 months to occur and about 3 months to clear after discontinuation of lens wear. They appear as round, transparent epithelia inclusions seen in reversed illumination. If the number of microcysts is more than 20 the lenses should be definitely replaced to ones with better oxygen transmissibility (Fig. 25.14).
2. Reduced nerve sensitivity.
3. Thinning of epithelium.

Fig. 25.14: Microcysts (*Courtsey:* IACLE)

4. *Epithelial injury:* Aberrations are common with rigid lenses, and happen wherever the tear exchange is hampered. It is also common to find SPK and superior arcuate lesion with soft lenses.
5. *Reduction in epithelial adhesion:* Chronic hypoxia leads to reduced epithelial adhesion due to decrease in hemidesmosomes synthesis. This may lead to pealing of the epithelium like an intact sheet from the cornea.
6. *Infiltrates:* Epithelial/subepithelial infiltrates are collection of lymphocytes that occur as a result of irritation from chemical preservatives and contaminated lenses.

Effect on Stroma

Edema (Striae and Folds) (Fig. 25.15)

The cornea swells as a result of increased accumulation of fluid in the stroma. This happens due to lack of oxygen, mechanical effects. Chronic levels of corneal edema results in adverse effects on corneal structure and function. Hypoxia leads to stromal edema. Striae and folds are the warning signs seen in stroma.

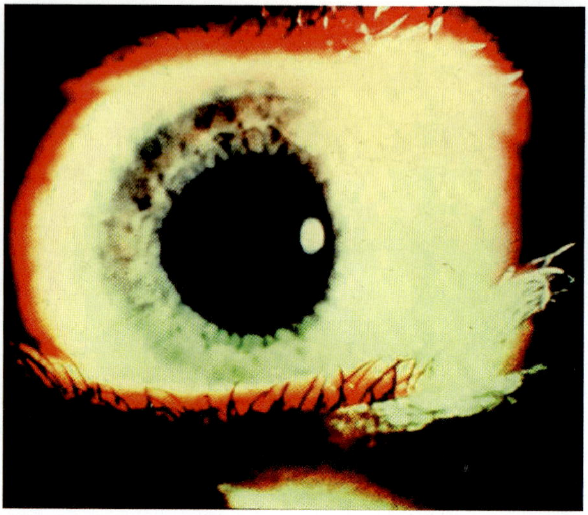

Fig. 25.15: Central corneal clouding (*Courtsey:* IACLE)

Stromal Thinning

The stroma if is subjected to hypoxia will lead to increase in osmolarity, reduction in pH and localized pressure. These changes lead to stromal edema that in turn leads to loss of GAGs. The loss of GAGs leads to stromal thinning. This means the true edema = apparent edema + stromal thinning.

Vascularization

Stromal keratocytes are associated with new vessel growth in the stroma. This happens as a result of chronic hypoxia. This is more common with hydrogels especially low water thick lenses, or high power lenses and extended wear. Vascularization is very less likely with rigid lenses.

Corneal Distortion

This is because of the biodegradation of the Bowman's membrane. Flat fitting rigid lenses create an orthokeratology effect. This was very common with PMMA lenses.

Effect on Endothelium

Polymegathesim is increase in cell size and *pleomorphism* is variation in cell size. Long-term chronic hypoxia leads to changes in endothelium cells. The barrier system of endothelium still remains unaffected. The trend to reversal is also insignificant on lens withdrawal. This happened more with PMMA and EW soft lenses. These changes are very less likely to happen with RGP lenses (Fig. 25.16).

Endothelial Blebs (Fig. 25.17)

They are a rapid response to low oxygen transmissibility lenses. They happen as early as in 30 minutes.

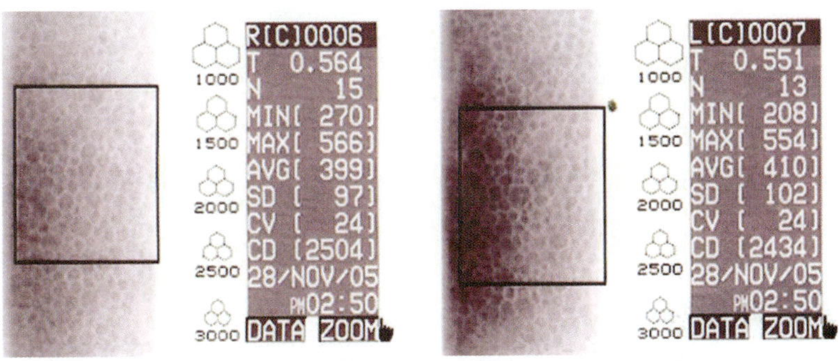

Fig. 26.16: Endothelial count

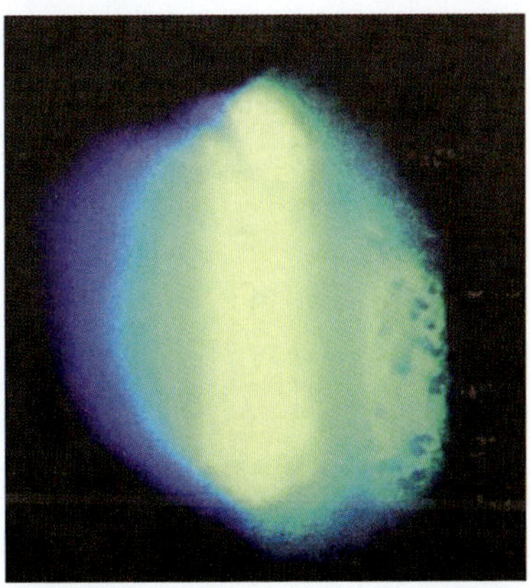

Fig. 25.17: Blebs (*Courtsey:* IACLE)

Appendices

Appendix 1: Diopters to radius of curvature conversion table

D R	D R	D R	D R	D R	D R	D R
36.00-9.37	39.00-8.65	42.00-8.03	45.00-7.50	48.00-7.03	51.00-6.61	54.00-6-25
36.12-9.33	39.12-8.62	42.12-8.01	45.12-7.48	48.12-7.01	51.12-6.60	54.12.6.23
36.25-9.30	39.25-8.59	42.25-7.98	45.25-7.45	48.25-6.99	51.25-6.58	54.25-6.22
36.37-9.27	39.37-8.57	42.37-7.96	42.37-7.43	48.37-6.97	51.37-6.56	54.37-6.20
36.50-9.24	39.50-8.54	42.50-7.94	42.50-7.41	48.50-6.95	51.50-6.55	54.50-6.19
36.62-9.21	39.62-8.51	42.62-7.91	42.62-7.39	48.62-6.94	51.62-6.53	54.62-6.17
36.75-9.18	39.75-8.49	42.75-7.89	42.75-7.37	48.75-6.92	51.75-6.52	54.75-6.16
36.87-9.15	39.87-8.45	42.87-7.87	42.87-7.35	48.87-6.90	51.87-6.50	54.87-6.15
37.00-9.12	40.00-8.43	43.00-7.84	46.00-7.33	49.00-6.88	52.00-6.49	55.00-6.13
37.12-9.09	40.12-8.41	43.12-7.82	46.12-7.31	49.12-6.87	52.12-6.47	55.00-6.12
37.25-9.06	40.25-8.38	43.25-7.80	46.25-7.29	49.25-6.85	52.25-6.46	55.00-6.10
37.37-9.03	40.37-8.36	43.37-7.78	46.37-7.27	49.37-6.83	52.37-6.44	55.00-6.09
37.50-9.00	40.50-8.33	43.50-7.75	46.50-7.25	49.50-6.81	52.50-6.42	55.00-6.08
37.62-8.97	40.62-8.30	43.62-7.73	46.62-7.23	49.62-6.80	52.62-6.41	55.00-6.06
37.75-8.94	40.75-8.28	43.75-7.71	46.75-7.21	49.75-6.78	52.75-6.39	55.00-6.05
37.87-8.91	40.87-8.25	43.87-7.69	46.87-7.20	49.87-6.76	52.87-6.38	55.00-6.04
38.00-8.88	41.00-8.23	44.00-7.67	47.00-7.18	50.00-6.75	53.00-6.36	
38.12-8.65	41.12-8.20	44.12-7.64	47.12-7.16	47.12-7.73	53.12-6.35	
38.25-8.82	41.25-8.18	44.25-7.62	47.25-7.14	47.25-7.71	53.25-6.33	
38.37-8.79	41.37-8.15	44.37-7.60	47.37-7.12	47.37-7.70	53.37-6.32	
38.59-8.76	41.59-8.13	44.59-7.58	47.59-7.10	47.59-7.68	53.59-6.30	
38.62-8.73	41.62-8.10	44.62-7.56	47.62-7.08	47.62-7.66	53.62-6.29	
38.75-8.70	41.75-8.08	44.75-7.54	47.75-7.06	47.75-7.65	53.75-6.27	
38.87-8.68	41.87-8.06	44.87-7.52	47.87-7.05	47.87-7.63	53.87-6.26	

Appendix 2: Vertex distance table: (13 mm vertex distance)

For minus (–) read right to left and for plus (+) read left to right			
5.00 = 4.75	8.00 = 7.37	12.75 = 11.00	20.00 = 16.50
5.12 = 4.87	8.12 = 7.50	13.00 = 11.25	21.00 = 17.50
5.37 = 5.00	8.25 = 7.62	13.50 = 11.50	22.00 = 17.50
5.50 = 5.12	8.50 = 7.75	13.75 = 11.75	23.00 = 18.00
5.62 = 5.25	8.75 = 8.00	14.00 = 12.00	24.00 = 18.50
5.75 = 5.37	9.00 = 8.25	14.25 = 12.25	24.50 = 19.00
5.87 = 5.50	9.25 = 8.37	14.75 = 12.50	25.50 = 19.50
6.00 = 5.62	9.50 = 8.62	15.00 = 12.75	26.00 = 20.00
6.12 = 5.75	9.75 = 8.75	15.50 = 13.00	27.50 = 21.00
6.37 = 5.87	10.00 = 9.00	15.75 = 13.25	28.50 = 22.00
6.50 = 6.00	10.25 = 9.12	16.25 = 13.50	30.00 = 23.00
6.62 = 5.25	10.50 = 9.25	16.75 = 13.75	31.00 = 24.50
6.75 = 5.37	10.75 = 9.37	17.00 = 14.00	23.00 = 25.00
6.87 = 5.50	11.00 = 9.62	17.25 = 14.25	35.00 = 26.50
7.00 = 5.62	11.25 = 9.75	17.62 = 14.37	38.00 = 27.00
7.12 = 5.75	11.50 = 10.00	18.00 = 14.50	41.00 = 28.00
7.37 = 5.87	11.75 = 10.25	18.12 = 14.75	43.00 = 29.00
7.50 = 6.00	12.00 = 10.37	18.50 = 15.00	45.00 = 30.00
7.62 = 5.25	12.50 = 10.75	18.75 = 15.25	
7.75 = 5.37		19.00 = 15.50	
7.87 = 5.50		19.50 = 16.50	

Appendix 3: Soft contact Lens—FDA Groups

Group 1 Low water (< 50% H_2O) Nonionic Polymers	*Group 2 High water (>50% H_2O) Nonionic Polymers*	*Group 3 Low water (< 50% H_2O) Ionic Polymers*	*Group 4 High water (> 50% H_2O) Ionic Polymers*
Tefilcon (38%) (Dk = 8) • Clbasoft • Cibathin • Torisoft • Softint • Bi-Soft • STD • Illusions	**Iodofilcon B (79%) (Dk = 38)** • CW 79 • LL 79	**Bufilcon A (45%) (Dk = 12)** • Hydrocurve II 45 • Soft Mate	**Bufilcon A (79%) (Dk = 16)** • Hydrocurve II • Hydrocurve II 55 bifocal
	Surfilcon (74%) (Dk = 35 • Permaflex	**Deltafilcon A (43%) (Dk = 10)** • Almsoft • Amsoft thin • Comfort Flex • Custom Flex • Metrosoft • Soft Form Toric	**Perfilcon (71%) (Dk = 34)** • Permalens • Permalens XL • Permalens Therapeutic
Tetrafilcon A (43%) (DK = 9) • AOSoft • Quaflex stanrdad • Aquaflex super thin • Ventage thin • Preference • Preference toric • Copper clear • Copper toric	**Lidofilcon A (70%) (Dk = 31)** • LL 70 • CV 70 • Q&E 70 • N&E 70	**Deoxifilcon A (47%) (Dk 17)** • Accugel	**Etafilcon A (58%) (Dk = 28)** • Acuvue • Surevue • 1-Day Acuvue **Ocufilcon B (53%) (Dk = 16)** • Ocu-flex • Continental

Contd...

Contd...

Group 1 Low water ($< 50\% H_2O$) Nonionic Polymers	*Group 2 High water ($>50\% H_2O$) Nonionic Polymers*	*Group 3 Low water ($< 50\% H_2O$) Ionic Polymers*	*Group 4 High water ($> 50\% H_2O$) Ionic Polymers*
Crofilcon (38%) (Dk = 12) • CSI clarity • CSI clarity toric • Aztech	**Netrafilcon A (65%)** • Gentle touch	**Phemfilcon A (38%) (Dk = 8)** • DuraSoft 2 • DuraSoft 2 Optifit	**Ocufilcon C (55%) (Dk = 16)** • UCL 55
Hefilcon A and B (50% (Dk = 12) • Flexlens • Unilens • Optima toric • Simulvue • Gold medialist toric	**Hefilcon C** • Gold Medialist Toric	**Ocufilcon (44%) (Dk = 16)** • Tresoft • Tresoft Thin	**Phemfilcon A (55%) (Dk = 16)** • DuraSoft 3 • DuraSoft 3 Optifit
Isofilcon (36%) (Dk = 5) • AL-47 **Isofilcon (33%) (Dk = 4)** • Menicon **Isofilcon (33%) (Dk = 4)**	**Alfafilcon A (66%) (Dk = 32)** • Softens 66 **Omafilcon A (59%) (Dk = 32)** • Proclear		**Methafilcon A (55%) (Dk = 18)** • Edge III 55 • Eclipse • Kontur • LL 55 • Metro 55 • SunFLex • Horizon 55 Bi-Con • Sunsoft Toric 15.0 • Westcon Toric and Sphere • Biocurve Toric and sphere

Contd...

Contd...

Group 1 Low water (< 50% H_2O) Nonionic Polymers	*Group 2 High water (>50% H_2O) Nonionic Polymers*	*Group 3 Low water (< 50% H_2O) Ionic Polymers*	*Group 4 High water (> 50% H_2O) Ionic Polymers*
• CustoEyes 38 • Softics • Allvue • Cellusoft • Hydron Mini • Hydron Zero • Hydron Toric • Hydron Zero T • Cooper Thin • LL38 • Ideal Soft • PS-45 Multifocal • Horizon 38 • Westfin Toric • Soft-form II • Soflens • EpconSOFT • Nuview • Soft view • Metrosoft II • Edge III • Edge III XT • Edge III Thin • Optima 38 • Ultra Flex • SeeQuence • Optima FW • Occasions multifocal			• LifeStyle frequency • Hydrosoft Toric and sphere **Methafilcon B (55%) (Dk = 16)** • Hydrasoft • Hydrasoft toric **Vifilcon A (55%) (DK = 16)** • Softcon • Softcon EW • Spectrum • Spectrum Toric • Spectrum bifocal • Newvues • Focus • Focus Toric

Index